Challenging Cases in

Pediatric Infectious Diseases

Volume 1

Keith R. Powell, MD, FAAP

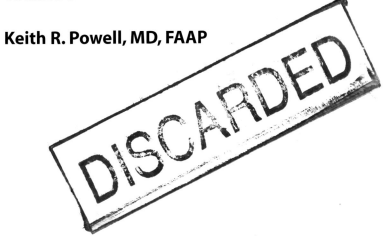

D1610691

American Academy of Pediatrics
141 Northwest Point Blvd
Elk Grove Village, IL 60007-1098

Editor: Martha Cook
Marketing Manager: Linda Smessaert
Production Manager: Theresa Wiener
Designer: Linda Diamond
Copy Editor: Jason Crase

Library of Congress Control Number 2005927506
ISBN-13: 978-1-58110-185-0
ISBN-10: 1-58110-185-6
MA0338

The recommendations in this publication do not indicate an exclusive course of treatment
or serve as a standard of care. Variations, taking into account individual circumstances,
may be appropriate.

Brand names are furnished for identification purposes only. No endorsement of the
manufacturers or products listed is implied.

9-153/0906

Printed in China

1 2 3 4 5 6 7 8 9 10

Table of Contents

Part 4
Case Reports in Teenagers

Acknowledgments

Challenging Cases in Pediatric Infectious Diseases could not have been written without support, motivation, encouragement, and help. William Considine, president and CEO of Akron Children's Hospital, supported my efforts and made it possible for me to work off campus where I could write with little interruption. Lori Lothian, a special person in my life, provided encouragement and companionship while I was writing in Vancouver. My children, Lindsey and Thomas, encouraged me to pass on some of what I have learned "for the children." Martha Cook, my editor, promised to help and came through in spades. I thank George Nankervis, MD, PhD; Blaise Congeni, MD; and John Bower, MD, for permission to use their wonderful picture collection. Finally, I deeply appreciate Owen Hendley, MD; John Bower, MD; and Blaise Congeni, MD, for their critical review and keeping me honest and more importantly, accurate. My gratitude to all.

Part 1

Case Reports in Newborns and Infants

Chapter 1

Fever and Facial Swelling 1

Presentation

A 6-month-old infant girl arrives in your office with a 1-day history of fever and a red, swollen right cheek (Figure 1). She was born at term and has been healthy until today. No one in the family is ill. The infant does receive care in a home child care setting, but none of the other children in child care are ill. Well-child care has been sporadic and the patient has not received any immunizations by choice of the parents. Physical examination reveals a well-developed, well-nourished 6-month-old who is alert and active, albeit fussy. Her temperature is 39.1°C (102.4°F); pulse, respiration, and blood pressure results are normal. The findings of her physical examination are normal except for swelling and a dusky purple discoloration of her left cheek (Figure 1). The skin over her left cheek is warm to touch. Preauricular or cervical lymphadenitis is absent. Tympanic membranes are normal.

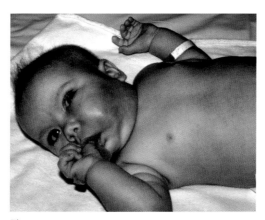

Figure 1

- **What is your differential diagnosis?**

- **How will you evaluate this patient?**

- **How will you treat the patient's condition?**

Discussion

Diagnosis

The differential diagnosis is limited. The acute onset of fever with discoloration, swelling, and warmth of the buccal mucosa puts buccal cellulitis at the top of your list. *Haemophilus influenzae* type b (Hib) was the most common cause of buccal cellulitis before universal immunization against Hib. Most cases occur in infants 6 months to 2 years of age. Ipsilateral acute otitis media has been reported in 32% to 67% of infants with buccal cellulitis. Oral mucosal lesions also have been reported in patients with buccal cellulitis, but others have not observed this finding. Neither otitis nor mucosal lesions are found in all infants with buccal cellulitis, leaving the pathogenesis speculative. More than half of infants with buccal cellulitis will be bacteremic with Hib; infants without overt signs have been found to have meningitis when a lumbar puncture was performed. Although the causative organism of buccal cellulitis in the vast majority of cases is Hib, *Streptococcus pneumoniae, Streptococcus agalactiae,* and *Staphylococcus aureus* also have been isolated from patients with indistinguishable clinical findings.

Popsicle panniculitis can occur when a popsicle is left in the mouth of an infant long enough to cause cold injury. The swelling and discoloration usually is closer to the corner of the mouth and the infant is afebrile and otherwise well (Figure 2). Frostbite (chilblains) is characterized by a doughy swelling and local cyanosis in areas exposed to the cold (Figure 3). Frostbite is more likely to involve both cheeks, while buccal cellulitis is almost always unilateral. Other symptoms of frostbite might include itching, burning, or pain, but there is no fever or systemic signs of illness.

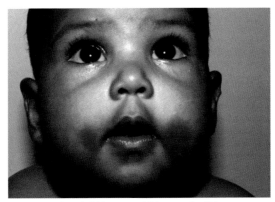

Figure 2. This child has popsickle panniculitis.
(Courtesy of Howard J. Bennett, MD, George
Washington University School of Medicine)

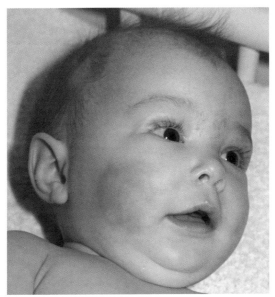

Figure 3. This child has frostbite (chilblains).
(Courtesy of Robert J. Giusti, MD, Long Island College
Hospital)

An insect bite or sting on the cheek could also cause acute swelling and erythema in the area surrounding the bite. Again, the infant would not be febrile or systemically ill.

This child has not been immunized; you are most worried about Hib buccal cellulitis and bacteremia. You order a CBC, differential count, and blood culture and give intramuscular ceftriaxone. You then call the emergency department of the local hospital, alert them of the infant's pending arrival, and ask them to perform a lumbar puncture.

The CBC shows a WBC count of 22,500 cells/µL with 65% granulocytes. The lumbar puncture has 2 WBCs with normal protein and glucose concentrations. The patient's oral intake was adequate, so you elect to continue to administer intramuscular ceftriaxone once daily. *Haemophilus influenzae* type B is isolated from the infant's blood, but culture of her cerebrospinal fluid was sterile. By the second day of hospitalization the patient is afebrile and the swelling in her cheek is resolving. The blood isolate was susceptible to ampicillin and you discharge the patient on oral amoxicillin to complete a total of 10 days of antibacterial therapy. You suggest that the family reconsider vaccination for their children.

Buccal cellulitis can be defined as warmth, tenderness, swelling, red or purple discoloration, and induration of the soft tissues of the cheek without evidence of an adjacent skin lesion. In a study of 72 patients with buccal cellulitis seen in Oklahoma, Ohio, and Alabama, patients ranged from 1.5 to 64 months of age with a median age of 11 months. The ratio of males to females was equal and the racial distribution of patients corresponded to the distribution of races in the 3 communities. Cases occurred throughout the year, but were more common in the fall and winter. The right cheek was involved twice as often as the left cheek. Otitis media was present in 38% of the patients and it was on the same side as the buccal cellulitis in 32% of patients. Fever and swelling of the cheek was present for fewer than 24 hours before hospitalization in two thirds of the patients (range of 4 hours to 5 days). Blood cultures were positive for Hib in 55% of the patients and 3 patients had Hib meningitis.

Treatment

Patients who do not have meningitis should receive 48 hours of parenteral antibacterial therapy followed by an oral antibacterial agent to complete a total of 7 to 10 days of therapy. Because Hib are often β-lactamase positive, a third-generation cephalosporin such as ceftriaxone or cefotaxime should be given parenterally. If a bacterial pathogen is not isolated, oral amoxicillin plus clavulanic acid can be given to cover β-lactamase–positive Hib.

Keep in Mind

The incidence of buccal cellulitis has diminished greatly since the institution of universal immunization against Hib in infancy. When you see a patient with buccal cellulitis, obtain an accurate immunization history, consider other pathogens, and remember that no vaccine is 100% effective.

Chapter 2

Papulopustular Rash

Presentation

You are seeing newborns at the local hospital before office hours. One of your patients is still in the hospital on day 5 of life because of maternal complications following cesarean delivery. She is scheduled to be discharged today. Instead of sending the baby home, you transfer him to the special care nursery. The reason for your concern is a widespread, splotchy red rash involving his face, trunk, and extremities (Figure 1).

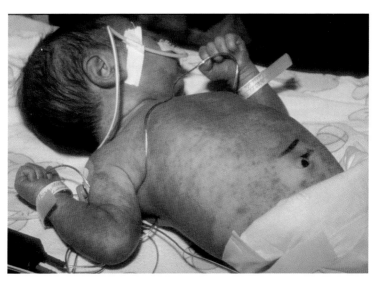

Figure 1

On closer inspection you see numerous pustular lesions with an erythematous base (Figure 2) and areas where papules and pustules are confluent.

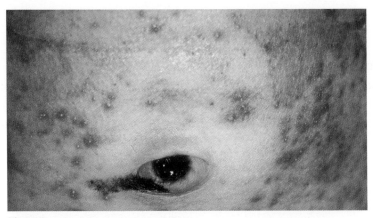

Figure 2

You talk to the mother and one of the nurses and learn that yesterday the baby had several scattered yellow-white lesions that were firm with a red base. The rash progressed over the next 24 hours. The newborn does not have a fever and his temperature has been stable. Mother is breastfeeding and it is not clear what his intake has been, but he has a good suck and has been at the breast about every 2 hours. He is voiding well and has passed meconium. The findings from the physical examination are normal except for the rash.

- **What is your differential diagnosis?**
- **How will you evaluate this newborn?**
- **How will you treat this newborn?**

Discussion

Diagnosis

The appearance of the rash makes you consider pyoderma, herpes simplex, candidiasis, and more benign conditions such as miliaria and erythema toxicum. You obtain material from the pustules for direct fluorescent antibody staining for herpes simplex virus, bacterial culture, and examination with Gram and H and E stains.

You call the laboratory and ask them to prepare the stained slides and perform the fluorescent antibody test for herpes simplex as soon as possible. Within 15 minutes the stained slides are ready for viewing; you go to the laboratory to look at them. The gram-stained specimen shows many neutrophils, but neither you nor the laboratory technician sees any bacteria or fungal forms. At the hematology station the laboratory technician shows you the H and E stained slide, which is loaded with eosinophils. You head back to the microbiology section of the laboratory and the technician tells you that the direct fluorescent antibody test result for herpes is negative. When you return to the special care nursery the baby's condition is unchanged.

You are feeling more comfortable that the neonate does not have a serious bacterial, fungal, or viral infection based on the preliminary laboratory findings and the stability of the neonate. Nonetheless, you call the neonatal intensive care unit and ask the neonatologist on service to come to the special care nursery and see the baby in case something changes and the baby needs intensive care. The neonatologist is able to examine the baby right away, so you wait to discuss the case with her. Despite the extensive rash and pustular nature, the neonatologist is confident the baby has erythema toxicum. The neonatologist tries to make you feel better by saying the negative laboratory results bolster this diagnosis; however, given the age of the baby (5 days), distribution, and appearance in an otherwise well newborn, a simple Wright stain of a lesion would have been sufficient to make the diagnosis.

Erythema toxicum is a benign, self-limited, evanescent rash that occurs in as many as half of all full-term newborns. Preterm newborns are not affected as often, but may have the onset of rash in the days or weeks after birth.

The baby does well over the next 24 hours and the mother tells you that the rash seems to wax and wane. It looks less impressive today than yesterday. Culture of the material from one of the pustules is not growing any bacteria. You discharge the baby and tell the mother the rash may continue to wax and wane for several days, but will gradually go away. It does.

Keep in Mind
The cause of erythema toxicum is not known, but the best way to make the diagnosis if the clinical diagnosis is uncertain is to stain for eosinophils. The condition runs its course quickly and no therapy is required.

Chapter 3

Bullous Lesions

Presentation

You are on service at your local hospital and you are asked to see a neonate for whom a primary care physician has not been identified. The 2-day-old newborn has bright red skin and multiple, bullous lesions (Figure). The mother, a teenager from Haiti, was the victim of a rape that occurred in Haiti. She received no prenatal care before delivering in the United States. You collect fluid from one of the bullae to send for culture and prescribe methicillin, thinking the infant has Ritter disease (staphylococcal scalded skin syndrome in a neonate) or bullous impetigo.

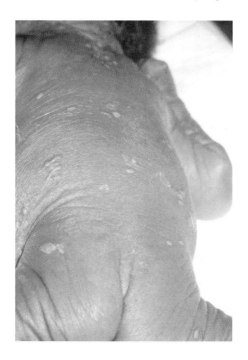

- ■ **What else should be in the differential diagnosis?**

- ■ **What tests would you order?**

- ■ **What follow-up care do you offer to this mother and her baby?**

Discussion

Diagnosis

The lack of prenatal care and history of rape raise great concern that the baby might have congenital syphilis. Nonetheless, the skin appears so much like scalded skin that you believe the history might be a red herring. After writing the order for methicillin you take a look at the mother's medical record. A quantitative nontreponemal antibody test, or venereal disease research laboratory (VDRL) slide test, was performed; the result is positive. You call the microbiology laboratory and ask them if they do dark-field examinations for *Treponema pallidum.* The answer is yes; they offer to obtain a specimen of fluid from one of the infant's bullous lesions.

You are back in your office when an excited laboratory technician calls to tell you the dark-field examination is positive for spirochetes; a Gram stain on the same specimen did not reveal any other bacteria.

You call the resident in the nursery, who already knows the results of the dark-field examination, and ask her how she would like to proceed. She would like to obtain a VDRL slide test, a rapid plasma reagin test, or an automated reagin test (ART) and a treponemal test (fluorescent treponemal antibody absorption [FTA-ABS] or *T pallidum* particle agglutination). To determine whether the infant has neurosyphilis, the resident would also like to do a lumbar puncture and send cerebrospinal fluid (CSF) for the same treponemal and nontreponemal tests, as well as a cell count and differential and protein and glucose concentrations. She also recommends long-bone x-ray films to look for pathologic changes and a CBC with differential and platelet counts to evaluate for thrombocytopenia. You agree with this workup and ask her to get permission from the mother for human immunodeficiency virus (HIV) testing of her baby.

You remind the resident that in addition to universal precautions, everyone touching the baby should wear gloves until the baby has been treated for 24 hours. You also suggest that the methicillin be changed to penicillin. Next you call the obstetrician to let him know your findings and suggest that the mother be tested for other sexually transmitted diseases including HIV.

The VDRL and FTA-ABS results are positive in serum and CSF. The x-ray film of the long bones shows a single layer of periosteal calcification (diaphyseal periostitis) and sawtooth metaphyseal dystrophy. The patient is also slightly thrombocytopenic. You are relieved to learn that the HIV test result is negative in the mother and her baby.

The diagnosis is clear. The baby has congenital syphilis with neural involvement.

Treatment
You treat the baby with intravenous penicillin G for 10 days. Follow-up care is very important. This newborn should have careful follow-up evaluations at 1, 2, 3, 6, and 12 months of age. You should repeat the VDRL when the baby is 3 and 6 months of age and the CSF VDRL at the 6-month visit. The VDRL should decrease by the time the baby is 3 months old and should be nonreactive by 6 months of age if the baby was adequately treated. If the VDRL titer is increasing, the baby should receive a 10-day course of parenteral penicillin G. If the VDRL titer persists at the same level at the 6-month visit, the baby should be treated with a 10-day course of parenteral penicillin G and reevaluated at 12 months, including a lumbar puncture.

Keep in Mind
Syphilis is the great imitator. Most babies with congenital syphilis are asymptomatic and your first clue will be learning that the mother's non-treponemal antibody test result is positive. When caring for a newborn always check the mother's test results.

Chapter 4

Swollen Eyelid

Presentation

An infant arrives in your office with a swollen eye (Figure 1). Two days ago this 11-month-old boy fell and hit his head on the edge of the coffee table in his living room, resulting in a small laceration just below his right eyebrow. The cut stopped bleeding easily and the parents did not think it needed stitches. He had a black eye the next day, but otherwise appeared normal. Now, his eye is swollen shut and there is yellow, crusted matter on his eyelids and at the corner of his eye. He feels warm. His mother measured his temperature at 39°C (102.2°F) with a temporal artery thermometer.

You confirm the temperature and observe a small wound surrounded by erythema on the upper eyelid. There is no pus draining from the wound, and no pus is expressed when palpating near the wound. The upper and lower eyelids are swollen and matted together and have a purple hue. After gently soaking the eyelids with warm tap water and removing the crusted exudates, you are able to see that his bulbar conjunctiva is clear, he has a

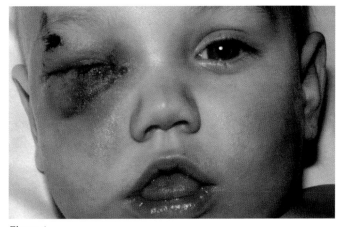

Figure 1

full range of ocular motion, and there is no chemosis or conjunctival hemorrhage. Neither Kernig nor Brudzinski signs are present. The findings of the remainder of his examination are normal.

- ■ **What is the differential diagnosis?**
- ■ **What information do you want to check in the medical record?**
- ■ **What tests do you want to obtain?**
- ■ **How will you treat this patient?**

Discussion

Diagnosis

Your first consideration is orbital cellulitis. However, because there is no proptosis, limitation of extraocular movements, or pain as he moves his eye, you feel comfortable that there is no involvement of retro-bulbar structures.

The next diagnosis you consider is periorbital cellulitis. You flip through his medical record and quickly determine that all of his immunizations are current, including 3 doses each of *Haemophilus influenzae* type b (Hib) and pneumococcal conjugate (PCV-7) vaccines. The immunization history makes infection with Hib or *Streptococcus pneumoniae* unlikely, but this could be group A β-hemolytic streptococcal (GABS) infection or *Staphylococcus aureus* infection of the wound with contiguous spread to the eyelids. The patient's age, the rapid onset of fever and swelling, and your concern about community-associated methicillin-resistant *S aureus* (CA-MRSA) leads you to hospitalize this boy for administration of parenteral antibacterial therapy. After admission to the infant unit the resident calls; you agree that specimens of blood and the exudate from the eye should be sent for culture and susceptibility testing.

The resident suggests intravenous vancomycin to treat CA-MRSA. You agree, but ask her to start ceftriaxone as well. It is more active against GABS and will provide treatment in case of infection caused by Hib, *S pneumoniae* (vaccine failure is possible), or *S pneumoniae* serotypes not included in PCV-7 vaccine.

The laceration and the black eye could be a sign of physical abuse, but you are not concerned because there are no other bruises, the story is a common one, and you have been this family's pediatrician for several years.

By the next morning the exudate is growing gram-positive cocci in clusters that are coagulase positive. The blood culture remains sterile. When you see your patient he is eating breakfast and his right eyelids, although still swollen, are partially open. The diagnosis is *S aureus* infection of the eyelids with the laceration as the portal of entry.

Treatment

You talk to the resident about discontinuing treatment with ceftriaxone and changing the antistaphylococci therapy. You decide to wait for the results of susceptibility testing before deciding on the best antibacterial because 70% of the community-acquired *S aureus* in your region are resistant to methicillin and 10% are resistant to clindamycin.

On hospital day 2 the swelling of the eyelids is almost gone. Susceptibility testing shows the isolate to be susceptible to clindamycin and trimethoprim-sulfamethoxazole. You discharge the patient on oral clindamycin to complete 7 days of antibacterial therapy.

Keep in Mind

Before Hib and PCV-7 vaccines were available, the majority of cases of periorbital cellulitis was caused by Hib, with pneumococci as the second most common cause (Figure 2). The bacteria infect the eyelids from the

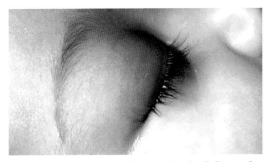

Figure 2. An infant girl with periorbital cellulitis and meningitis caused by *Haemophilus influenzae* type b.

blood or (more commonly in the case of *S pneumoniae)* the ethmoid sinuses via facial veins. Usually, GABS and staphylococcal infections start with a wound infection.

Orbital cellulitis is a sight-threatening infection and must be ruled out. If there is proptosis, decreased ocular motion, or orbital pain you should obtain a CT scan of the orbit. If you are not sure, consult a pediatric ophthalmologist.

Chapter 5

Waxy, Scaly, Itchy Rash

Presentation

This little girl comes to your office for a sick visit because she is fussy, especially at night, and has a rash that has worsened over the past couple of days (Figure 1). You have known this child since birth. She is growing and developing normally, is healthy, and is fully immunized for her age.

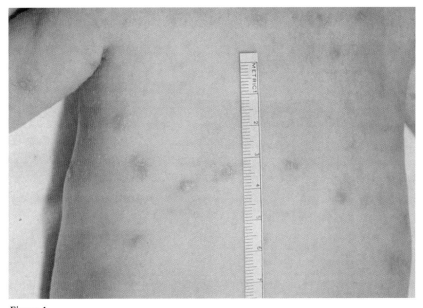

Figure 1

There are a few vesicles, but the rash is chiefly erythematous papules that have a waxy, scaly feel. Her whole body is involved (Figure 2), including her palms and soles (Figure 3). You look for threadlike tracks, but do not find any.

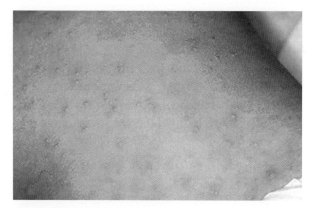

Figure 2

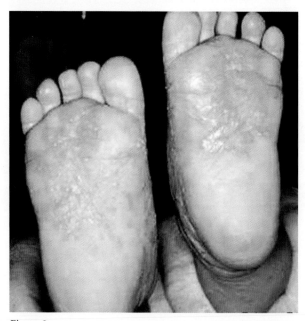

Figure 3

You ask the mother whether anyone else in the family has a similar rash. The mother says that no one has a rash that looks like the baby's, but that she has some very itchy sores on her hands (Figure 4).

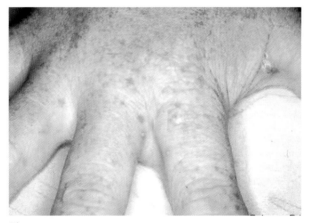

Figure 4

■ **What does this family have?**

■ **How will you treat the condition?**

Discussion

Diagnosis

The rash looks like a hypersensitivity reaction, but is too widespread to represent contact dermatitis. The rash does not look urticarial or infected. The distribution of the rash and history do not fit the diagnosis of eczema. There are lesions on the scalp, but it does not look like seborrhea (patients with severe seborrhea may have a secondary hypersensitivity dermatitis covering the body). The big clue in this case is the lesion between the mother's thumb and forefinger. You think this is most likely scabies.

It is a slow day in the office, so you grab some immersion oil and a scalpel and scrape one of the lesions on the mother's hand. You put the scrapings on a glass slide, drop on a cover slip, and examine the slide under low power (Figure 5). You call your partners to have a look at the *Sarcoptes scabiei* subspecies *hominis* mite that you have uncovered.

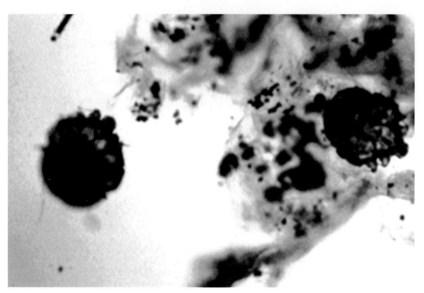

Figure 5

The adult female burrows in the upper layers of the epidermis, leaving serpiginous tracks followed by a papular, erythematous, and very pruritic eruption. Pruritus usually is worse at night. The rash is a hypersensitivity reaction to mite proteins and mite scybala (feces). In older children and adults the mites go for interdigital folds, flexor aspects of wrists, extensor surfaces of elbows, anterior axillary folds, the waistline, thighs, the navel, genitalia, areolae, the abdomen, the intergluteal cleft, and buttocks. In younger children, they will go anywhere. Sometimes you will see red-brown nodules on covered parts of the body such as the genitalia, groin, and axilla that can persist for months. These nodules (Figure 6) are a granulomatous response to dead mite antigens and scybala.

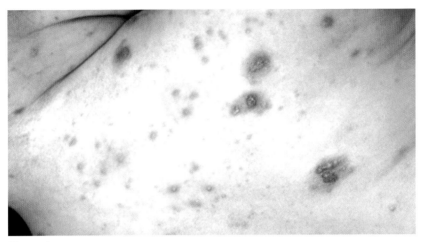

Figure 6

Treatment

The preferred drug for the treatment of scabies in infants and children is 5% permethrin cream. Lindane cream or lotion should be used only if other treatment options have failed. Crotamiton cream or lotion is an alternative. Infants and young children should receive whole-body treatment, while older children and adults can be treated from the neck down. Follow the manufacturer's instructions on the use of these agents. Because it may take as long as 2 months after contracting mites for scabies to appear, all household contacts should undergo prophylaxis at the same time the patient is treated.

Mites can live for 4 days only without benefit of a human host. All clothing and bedding that have been in contact with skin in the 4 days before treatment should be washed in hot water and dried using the high temperature setting. Articles that cannot be washed should be stored in a plastic bag for 4 days.

Keep in Mind

Scabies is a hypersensitivity reaction that may persist for several weeks after therapy. The major symptom is itching, which may be relieved by oral antihistamines or topical corticosteroids. As soon as treatment has been completed, children may return to child care or school.

Chapter 6

Pustular Lesions

Presentation

A 9-day-old newborn is in your office because her mother is concerned about 2 sores on the baby's back that she noticed while bathing her this morning. The neonate, born at term after an uncomplicated pregnancy, labor, and delivery, is doing well otherwise. You examined the patient at the birthing hospital on her first day of life and the findings of the examination were normal. The mother and baby were discharged from the hospital on the newborn's second day of life. The newborn is breastfeeding exclusively and has regained her birth weight.

On examination the baby is alert and fixes her gaze on you. She is afebrile and her vital signs are normal. She is 75th percentile for height, weight, and head circumference. Examination of the skin reveals only the 2 lesions on the neonate's back that the mother had noticed (figures 1 and 2).

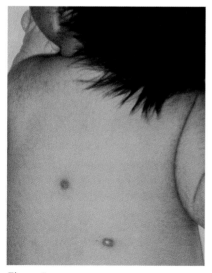
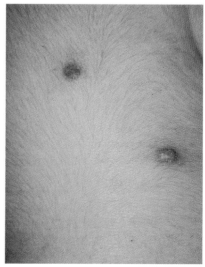

Figure 1

Figure 2

There is a vesiculopustular lesion to the left of the midline that is 3 to 4 mm in diameter and contains a yellowish fluid. There is a slight erythematous halo around the lesion. The second lesion has ruptured and a shallow ulcer with an erythematous base remains. Examination of the scalp is difficult because the newborn has a full head of hair. Nonetheless, you do not find any suspicious lesions on the scalp. Her eyes, ears, nose, and throat are normal. Results from examination of the heart and lungs are normal. Her liver and spleen are not enlarged and you do not feel an abdominal mass. She moves all of her extremities and has good grasp, Moro, sucking, startle, and rooting reflexes.

- **What is your differential diagnosis?**
- **What diagnostic tests will you perform?**
- **What treatment do you initiate?**

Discussion

Diagnosis

The neonate appears so healthy that your first impulse is to attribute these lesions to a superficial staphylococcal infection and treat her with a topical antibacterial agent. However, you are also aware that this is the age at which neonatal herpes skin lesions can arise. You ask the mother about herpes and she tells you that she has had fever blisters in the past, but the last one was several years ago. She is not aware of ever being exposed to or having genital herpes. Her husband does not, to her knowledge, have genital herpes, and she has been monogamous during their 6-year courtship and marriage. You explain your concern to the mother and tell her that you would like to have the baby seen by the pediatric infectious disease specialist before the second lesion ruptures, if that is possible. The mother agrees; you call an ID specialist and tell her your concerns. She asks you to send the patient directly to the emergency department (ED) so that she can see the lesions and obtain an appropriate specimen for diagnostic evaluation.

The patient arrives at the ED with the vesiculopustular lesion intact. The ID specialist confirms the history and physical examination. She then unroofs the intact lesion with a sterile needle, collects the fluid, and vigorously rubs the base of the lesion with a polyethylene terephthalate fiber swab. The specimen on the swab is sent for herpes simplex virus (HSV) culture and direct fluorescent antibody stain. The rapid direct immunofluorescent staining is diagnostic for HSV type 2. This is confirmed by subsequent culture results.

Although congenital HSV infections occur, the vast majority of cases of neonatal herpes are acquired from the birth canal during vaginal delivery. It is estimated that about 1 newborn per 3,000 births will be infected. There are no signs or symptoms of herpes infection at the time of delivery in 70% to 80% of mothers whose babies are infected in the birth canal, and the history for herpes is negative in the majority of cases. Signs and symptoms of infection in the neonate occur between 7 and 14 days after birth, with most cases occurring between 9 and 11 days after birth. Approximately 80% of newborns with neonatal herpes will have skin lesions. In one study, skin vesicles alone were the presenting sign in 40 of 56 newborns with neonatal herpes, but 28 of the newborns who presented with skin lesions alone had progressive disease. Four developed eye involvement, 9 developed localized central nervous system (CNS) disease, and 15 developed disseminated disease. You should not be too reassuring to the parents of a newborn who has only skin lesions at the time of presentation.

There are 3 clinical presentations of neonatal herpes infection, each occurring in about one third of infected newborns. Skin, eye, and mouth (SEM) involvement is the least severe. In a large collaborative treatment study, none of the neonates with SEM involvement died. However, neonates with SEM involvement who have 3 or more recurrences in the 6 months following diagnosis are at risk for neurologic impairment despite therapy.

The second type of presentation is CNS infection, including focal encephalitis and meningoencephalitis. These neonates have a fever and decreased level of consciousness and progress to having seizures that may be focal and difficult to control. Analysis of cerebrospinal fluid will show a mildly decreased glucose concentration, elevated protein concentration, and predominantly mononuclear cell pleocytosis (50–100 WBC). The mortality

rate for newborns with CNS herpes infection is about 15% and survivors
are likely to have significant neurologic sequelae.

The third type of presentation of neonatal herpes infection is disseminated
infection that can involve multiple organs including the liver, lungs, brain,
skin, and adrenal glands. The clinical findings include respiratory insufficiency, vascular instability, bleeding, hepatomegaly, and neurologic deterioration. The mortality rate for disseminated disease is 25% or greater despite
aggressive antiviral therapy. Newborns who present with SEM involvement
can progress to having CNS or disseminated disease.

A lumbar puncture should be performed on all neonates even if the only
sign of disease is skin lesions. The CSF should be cultured for herpes in
addition to being tested for herpes using the polymerase chain reaction
(PCR). Polymerase chain reaction is specific and more sensitive than culture, although not 100% sensitive. Seven of 29 neonates with only skin, eye,
or mouth lesions who were enrolled in a national collaborative study of the
treatment of neonatal herpes infections had herpes DNA in their spinal
fluid as detected by PCR. Protein, glucose, and cell counts were normal in
these 7 infants and culture of the CSF was negative for herpes. Five of the 6
infants who were evaluated at 12 months of age were developing normally,
while one had microcephaly, hypertonia, and developmental delay.

Treatment
All newborns with neonatal herpes infection should be treated with intravenous acyclovir. Infants with SEM involvement who have CSF that is
negative for herpesvirus by PCR can be treated for 14 days. All other newborns should receive 21 days of parenteral therapy. Disease may recur after
treatment; the optimal treatment of recurrences is unknown. The role of
long-term or intermittent suppressive therapy to prevent CNS sequelae
in neonates with SEM involvement also is not known, but it is under
investigation.

Keep in Mind

Herpes simplex skin lesions on neonates can look like vesicles, impetigo, or bullae. Always think about herpes when newborns have suspicious-looking lesions during the first 4 weeks of life. The medical history is not reliable in identifying babies at risk.

Chapter 7

Diaper Rash

Presentation

A young father brings his firstborn to your office for his 2-month well-child visit and is most concerned about the baby's diaper rash, which first appeared 2 days ago and is worsening. This infant was born at term and has been well. He received a birth dose of hepatitis B virus vaccine and is due for his next round of immunizations today. Except for the diaper rash (Figure), the results of the physical examination are normal. The baby's scrotum, thigh creases, and perianal region are bright red and there are scattered red macules and pustules. The infant is breastfed exclusively and the parents use ultra-absorbent disposable diapers.

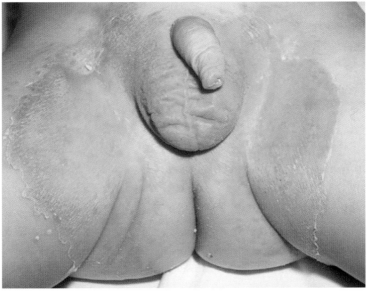

Figure (Courtesy of Daniel P. Krowchuk, MD, Wake Forest University School of Medicine, Winston-Salem, NC.)

- **What is your diagnosis?**

- **Will you order any tests?**

- **What treatment, if any, do you consider?**

Discussion

Diagnosis

The most common types of diaper rash are chafing dermatitis, *Candida* diaper dermatitis, atopic dermatitis, seborrheic dermatitis, and psoriasis. Chafing dermatitis appears only in the diaper area and is most prominent in areas where there is skin-to-skin friction such as the inner surface of the thighs, genitals, buttocks, and abdomen. The skin is slightly erythematous and has a shiny appearance. Occasionally papules will be present. Chafing dermatitis usually waxes and wanes quickly.

Candida diaper dermatitis usually becomes apparent after an infant has had a diaper rash for longer than 72 hours. Infection of the diaper rash with *Candida albicans* results in a confluent, intense red rash with well-demarcated borders. The distribution of the rash is the same as chafing dermatitis, but there are usually papules and pustules at the margin of the rash.

Infants with atopic dermatitis also can develop diaper dermatitis. This diagnosis is usually made by the presence of typical lesions of atopic dermatitis on the cheeks, neck, antecubital fossae, or extremities.

Infants with seborrheic dermatitis have a red, scaly rash that is most prominent in the thigh and gluteal creases. They also have similar lesions on their scalp, neck, trunk, or extremities.

Psoriasis is a much less common cause of diaper rash and is characterized by plaques of erythema with heavy scale in the diaper area, trunk, and scalp. There is usually a family history of psoriasis.

Most diaper dermatitis probably begins because of the high degree of moisture in the diaper area, which causes maceration of the skin. Friction and irritants from the stool and urine can then break down the surface of the epidermis, creating an environment favorable for growth of *C albicans*. The bright red erythema with satellite papules and pustules in this infant make *Candida* diaper dermatitis most likely. You advise the father to change diapers frequently, cleanse the diaper area with warm water at each change, and apply nystatin cream 4 times a day.

Treatment

Two placebo-controlled trials failed to show any benefit from giving oral nystatin in addition to topical nystatin. Until there is evidence to the contrary, topical therapy for uncomplicated *Candida* diaper dermatitis is sufficient. There is a large selection of topical antifungal agents to choose from, including topical nystatin, miconazole, clotrimazole, naftifine, ketoconazole, econazole, or ciclopirox. Nystatin is the least expensive of these drugs and usually is effective.

Keep in Mind

It has been estimated that 7% to 35% of the infant population in diapers has diaper dermatitis on any given day. It is unlikely that an infant will make it through the diaper-wearing stage without ever having a diaper rash.

Chapter 8

Fever and Facial Swelling 2

Presentation

An 11-month-old boy is due to arrive in your office for a sick visit. His mother called your office after discovering that the left side of the infant's face was bright red and swollen. The nurse reports that the infant was well last night, but when he awakened in the morning he was warm to touch and quite fussy. His mother measured his temperature rectally and it was 39.5°C (103.1°F). It was in the early afternoon that the mother noted the sudden onset of facial redness and swelling and called your office. You review the infant's medical record before he arrives and find that he is fully immunized for his age and has been well except for a moderately severe case of chickenpox when he was 8 months old. When you see the mother, you recall that she was in your office recently with her 9-year-old, who had streptococcal pharyngitis. The mother is quite upset. In the hour it has taken to travel to your office the patient's face has become more swollen and he has been crying in pain. You do not have to look very hard to see what she is concerned about (Figure 1).

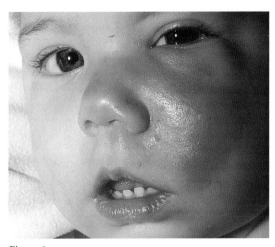

Figure 1

The left side of the boy's face from just above his upper lip to his lower eye-lid and from the middle of his nose to the lateral corner of his left eye is bright red and swollen. The center of the inflamed area has a rough appearance that looks like an orange peel, and the margins of the inflamed area are well demarcated. The skin is hot to touch and the patient cries when you palpate the inflamed area. There is no involvement of the eye and you do not see a scratch or anything that looks like a nidus for infection. His temperature is 40°C (104°F), pulse is 120 beats per minute, respiratory rate is 24 breaths per minute, and blood pressure is 90/60 mm Hg. Eyes, ears, nose, and throat are normal; there is no cervical adenopathy. The findings of the remainder of his examination are normal. Although the infant is stable and this process seems localized to the skin of his face, you are very concerned about the rapid progression.

You tell the mother to go directly to the local emergency department (ED), which is not even a 5-minute drive from the office, and you call the ED to tell the doctors that the mother is on her way with her infant.

- **What do you think this little boy has?**
- **What diagnostic tests would you like performed?**
- **How will you treat this patient?**

Discussion

Diagnosis
The redness, pain, warmth, swelling, well-demarcated margins, and location on the face lead you to believe this infant has erysipelas. The sibling with streptococcal pharyngitis provides a possible source for the infection. Alternatively, the patient's age and high fever can indicate bacterial sepsis. Herpes zoster is a possible diagnosis because the involved skin is in the same area as the distribution of the second division of the fifth cranial nerve (ophthalmic nerve) and the patient has a history of chickenpox. The

rapid onset, high fever, well-demarcated borders, and the absence of vesicles argue against zoster. Giant urticaria or contact dermatitis could possibly look like this, but the high fever and the absence of pruritus make these diagnoses unlikely. The distribution of the lesion is more cephalad than you would expect with *Haemophilus influenzae* type b (Hib) buccal cellulitis and the immunization status makes Hib infection unlikely, but not impossible. Staphylococcal infections usually do not progress this rapidly. You and the emergency medicine doctor agree that the patient probably has erysipelas caused by group A β-hemolytic streptococci (GABS). Nonetheless, the patient could have a staphylococcal or Hib infection, so you obtain blood for a CBC and to culture and a throat swab to culture and give intravenous ceftriaxone and vancomycin. The patient has remained stable in the ED and you decide to admit him to the general care unit.

The CBC shows WBC count of 15,200 cells/μL with a left shift.

Within 24 hours the patient is markedly improved. His temperature is almost normal, the swelling and redness of his face has diminished considerably, and he is no longer experiencing pain. The result from his blood culture is negative (only 5% of patients with erysipelas have positive results from blood cultures). His throat culture is positive for GABS. This is somewhat surprising because GABS is isolated from the throat in only 20% of patients with erysipelas.

Treatment
You change the patient's antibacterial therapy to oral penicillin V for 10 days and send him home.

Keep in Mind
Although erysipelas is primarily a clinical diagnosis, the disease may progress so rapidly that you will be concerned about other causes. For unknown reasons, erysipelas, which in the past most commonly involved

the face, now occurs on the legs in 80% of patients (Figure 2). Group A
β-hemolytic streptococcus infection seems to have cycles in which invasive
disease is more or less common. During those times when you see invasive
GABS disease, think of erysipelas.

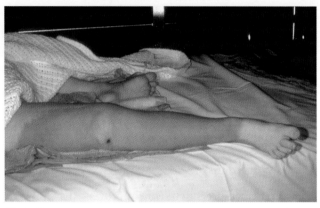

Figure 2

Chapter 9

Cat Scratch Wound

Presentation

Yesterday, this little boy met Aunt Ethyl's cat and ended up with some scratches on his face. (The cat fared much better.) This morning the child's eye is puffy and there is a serous exudate (Figure). His cheek is red, swollen, and warm to touch. His temperature is 38.2°C (100.8°F).

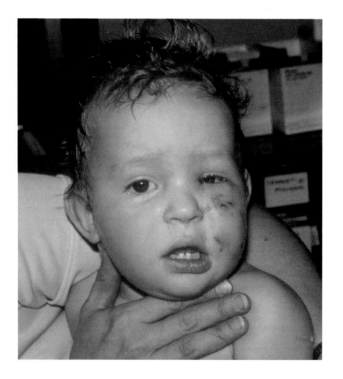

■ **What is the most likely pathogen causing this cellulitis?**

■ **How will you treat it?**

Discussion

Diagnosis

Approximately 70% to 90% of cats (and 25%–50% of dogs) carry *Pasteurella* species in their mouths, most commonly *Pasteurella multocida*. Of course, you must also consider *Staphylococcus aureus* and *Streptococcus pyogenes* (group A β-hemolytic streptococci [GABS]) when you have a patient with cellulitis.

You swab the exudate from one of the scratches and send the specimen for culture. Because the infection is on the face and has progressed quickly, you elect to hospitalize this little boy and start parenteral antibacterial agents.

The next morning the patient is afebrile and the redness, swelling, and warmth on his cheek have decreased. There is almost no eyelid swelling. The laboratory reports the growth of gram-negative coccobacilli, which are later identified as *P multocida*.

Treatment

P multocida is susceptible to penicillin, so it is a simple matter to treat GABS and *P multocida* with one drug. Treating a suspected case of *S aureus* and *Pasteurella* is a bit trickier. *Pasteurella* species are generally resistant to macrolides and clindamycin, and their susceptibility to β-lactams is variable. *Pasteurella* species are susceptible to amoxicillin, cefuroxime, cefpodoxime, trimethoprim-sulfamethoxazole, and doxycycline, but are resistant to cephalexin, cefadroxil, cefaclor, and dicloxacillin. Bite wound infections are frequently polymicrobial and there is an increasing incidence of community-associated methicillin-resistant staphylococci. Therefore, it is usually best to start with 2 antibacterials and modify therapy based on culture results. This patient was treated with penicillin and clindamycin and the clindamycin was stopped when only *P multocida* was isolated.

Keep in Mind

The susceptibility pattern of *Pasteurella* species is not intuitive; bite or scratch wound infections often have more than one pathogen. Use a reliable reference on susceptibility to begin therapy. After the susceptibility patterns of isolates from your patient are determined, make changes as necessary.

Be careful to exclude injury to the eyes following cat-inflicted wounds to the face. Corneal lacerations cannot be identified by fluorescein staining, so if there is any question of eye injury, consult an ophthalmologist.

Chapter 10

Fever and a Rash

Presentation

It is November and this 9-month-old infant arrives in your office because he has developed a rash (figures 1 and 2). He has had a fever for the past 4 or 5 days. He has been a little cranky when febrile, but resumes his usual behavior when his temperature is normal. His temperature measures as high as 40°C (104°F) each day, but he has been drinking well and eating adequately. He does not have any signs of an upper respiratory tract infection. You palpate some postauricular lymph nodes.

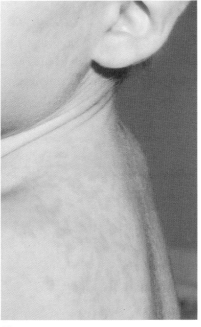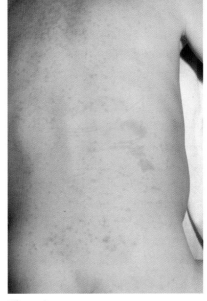

Figure 1   Figure 2

- **What is your differential diagnosis?**

- **Do you have a differential diagnosis?**

- **What will you tell the family?**

Discussion

Diagnosis

It is November and in your region of the country, enterovirus season is over. The patient has not been immunized for measles or rubella yet, but a nonspecific febrile illness for 4 to 5 days without a rash does not fit either disease. You consider a hypersensitivity reaction, but he is not on any medications and nothing new has been added to his diet. Again, the antecedent fever is not typical of hypersensitivity reactions. Roseola, or exanthema subitum of yore, is the most likely diagnosis.

Roseola is caused by human herpesvirus 6 (HHV-6) and occasionally by human herpesvirus 7 (HHV-7). The diagnosis of roseola is clinical; diagnostic tests for HHV-6 infections are available only in research laboratories. Only about 20% of children with a primary HHV-6 infection will develop a rash as they defervesce, allowing you to make the diagnosis. The rash may last for a few hours or 2 to 3 days. The vast majority of infants and children with primary HHV-6 infections have a nonspecific febrile illness that is characterized by temperatures in the 39.5°C (103.1°F) range for 3 to 7 days. Some children will have cervical or postauricular adenopathy or respiratory or gastrointestinal tract signs. Many children who are evaluated for suspected sepsis have HHV-6 infections. As many as 10% to 15% of infants evaluated in an emergency department for possible sepsis with a seizure were later found to have HHV-6 infections. It is not clear whether the seizures are simple febrile seizures or related to HHV-6 central nervous system infection.

The role of HHV-7 in roseola is less clear, but HHV-7 may account for second episodes of roseola. Like other herpesvirus infections, once infected with HHV-6 or HHV-7 you are always infected and can intermittently shed virus for life. Infectious virus can be isolated from the saliva of about 75% of adults. Thus, infants and children most likely become infected through contact with saliva of asymptomatic adult contacts. Maternally acquired antibody protects young infants for the first months of life. The peak incidence of HHV-6 infections is in infants and young children aged 6 to 24 months. Nearly all children are seropositive for HHV-6 by 4 years of age.

Treatment
The treatment of HHV-6 and HHV-7 infections is supportive.

Keep in Mind
A rash following a nonspecific febrile illness allows you to diagnose roseola and is very gratifying for you and reassuring to the family.

Chapter 11

Fever, Red Eyes, and Rash

Presentation

It is August and a 9-month-old infant boy is in your office for his second sick visit in 2 days. You initially saw him for fever and red eyes. His temperature on the first visit was 39°C (102.2°F) and his conjunctivae were injected (Figure 1). The findings of the remainder of his physical examination were normal. You suspected that he had viral conjunctivitis and recommended watchful waiting.

The mother calls the office on the sixth day of fever because her infant is very irritable, has a rash on his trunk, is not eating or drinking well, and

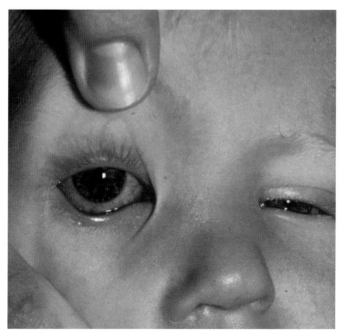

Figure 1

has bright red lips. You ask them to come to the office. On examination you find an ill-appearing infant who does not want to be touched. His rectal temperature is 39.2°C (102.6°F), respiratory rate is 22 breaths per minute, pulse is 96 beats per minute, and blood pressure is 100/70 mm Hg. His conjunctivae are almost clear, his lips and oral mucosa are bright red (Figure 2), and he has a strawberry tongue.

He has a non-tender polymorphous macular rash on his face and trunk (Figure 3). His lymph nodes are not enlarged. His hands and feet appear red and swollen (figures 4 and 5). The Kernig sign is positive.

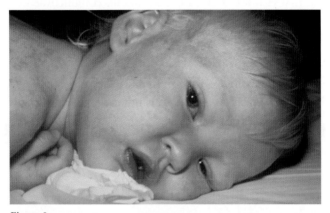

Figure 2

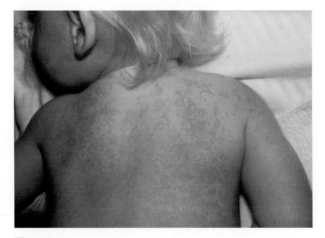

Figure 3

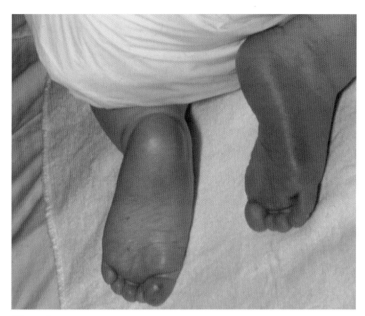

Figure 4

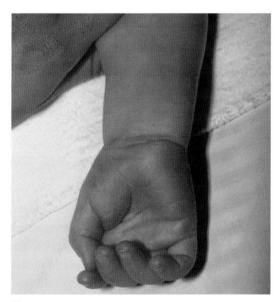

Figure 5

- ■ **What is your differential diagnosis?**

- ■ **What questions would you like to ask?**

- ■ **What diagnostic studies would you order?**

- ■ **What treatment would you recommend?**

Discussion

Diagnosis

The patient has many of the features of Kawasaki disease, but you know that group A streptococcal infection, toxic shock syndrome, enterovirus or adenovirus infection, Rocky Mountain spotted fever, Lyme disease, measles, leptospirosis, a connective tissue disease, or a drug reaction could have a similar appearance.

The history helps you narrow the differential diagnosis. The patient has not received measles vaccine, but the family has not left Ohio or been visited by anyone from outside of Ohio. Measles is extremely unlikely. It is August; although Lyme disease and Rocky Mountain spotted fever are very unlikely in Ohio, you ask about ticks and the mother says she has never seen any on this infant or anyone in the family. The mother says that there are no pets in the home and denies the possibility of her infant having been exposed to pond or creek water, making leptospirosis unlikely. Enterovirus infections are ubiquitous in August, but this patient does not attend child care and the mother is not aware of any sick contacts. You also note that the infant is not on any medications and the mother states that there are no drugs in the home that the boy could have been given.

Because of the positive Kernig sign and the infant's ill appearance, you refer him to the local emergency department for a lumbar puncture and further evaluation. The opening pressure is normal. The cerebrospinal fluid (CSF) has 90 WBC (all lymphocytes) and normal glucose and protein concentrations. The Gram stain result of the CSF is negative. Rapid strep test finding is negative, so a throat swab is sent for culture. A rapid test for adenovirus returns a negative result. A urinalysis shows 5 to 10 WBC per high power field, but no bacteria. The peripheral WBC count is 14,000 cells/μL with 60% polys and 15% bands. The platelet count is 320,000 platelets/μL.

With fever for 6 days, conjunctival injection, hyperemia of the oral mucosa, redness and swelling of the hands and feet, polymorphous rash, pyuria, and aseptic meningitis and no evidence for another disease, the most likely diagnosis is Kawasaki disease (mucocutaneous lymph node syndrome).

Treatment

The little boy is given 2 g/kg immunoglobulin intravenous (IGIV) and high-dose aspirin. Within 24 hours the rash is gone except for continued desquamation of the perineum. The infant is afebrile and much less irritable and his mucus membranes are not as red as at presentation.

You should begin therapy as soon as possible in patients in whom you suspect Kawasaki disease. When treatment is started 10 or more days after onset of illness, it is not known how effective the therapy will be at preventing coronary artery disease. Treatment should nonetheless be given if there are any signs of ongoing inflammation or evidence of coronary artery disease. Even with prompt treatment, 2% to 4% of patients will develop coronary artery abnormalities.

About 5% to 15% of patients who receive IGIV and aspirin therapy will have persistent or recurrent fever after being afebrile for 1 to 2 days. Many of these patients will benefit from a second dose of IGIV and continued high-dose aspirin therapy. Uncontrolled studies suggest that corticosteroid therapy may be beneficial in some patients who fail IGIV therapy. There are also case reports of patients with persistent arthritis or persistent or recrudescent fever who responded to treatment with a chimeric murine/human IgG1 monoclonal antibody (infliximab) that binds specifically to human tumor necrosis factor α-1.

After the patient has been afebrile for 4 to 5 days the high aspirin dose is lowered to a minimum daily low dose to maintain antithrombotic activity. If no coronary abnormalities are found by echocardiogram at 6 to 8 weeks following therapy, the aspirin may be discontinued.

The diagnosis of Kawasaki disease is made when a patient meets the case definition and other possible diagnoses have been excluded. The case definition requires fever for 5 days and at least 4 of the following 5 findings:

- Bilateral bulbar conjunctival injection
- Hyperemia of the oropharynx (ie, red pharynx, strawberry tongue, cherry red lips [may be dry and fissured])
- Redness or swelling of the hands and feet (Desquamation of the digits usually occurs after 10 days and is not helpful in making an initial diagnosis.)
- Rash (polymorphous can be maculopapular or morbilliform or resemble erythema multiforme) usually on the trunk and frequently more pronounced in the perineum
- Cervical lymphadenopathy

Lymphadenopathy is found in fewer than half of white children with Kawasaki disease. Symptoms commonly associated with Kawasaki disease include

- Marked irritability
- Abdominal pain
- Vomiting
- Diarrhea
- Urethritis with sterile pyuria
- Hepatic dysfunction
- Hydrops of the gallbladder
- Aseptic meningitis
- Pericardial effusion
- Arthritis (less common)
- Myocarditis (rarely)

Incomplete Kawasaki disease is a tricky diagnosis because by definition, patients do not meet the case definition for Kawasaki disease. Incomplete Kawasaki disease is most common in children younger than 1 year and should be considered when some of the clinical and laboratory findings suggest Kawasaki disease in a child who remains febrile for more than 7 days. If the child has been febrile for more than 7 days and you are considering the diagnosis of incomplete Kawasaki disease, an echocardiogram should be performed to look for coronary artery dilatation or aneurysm. If the echocardiogram is normal and your index of suspicion remains high, the patient should be given IGIV and high-dose aspirin within 10 days of onset of the fever.

About half of the cases of Kawasaki disease occur in children younger than 2 years and 80% occur in children younger than 5 years. The male-to-female ratio is about 1.5:1 and the incidence is highest in Asian Americans. The cause is not known and there is no evidence of person-to-person or common-source spread.

Complications
The major complication in children with Kawasaki disease is coronary artery aneurysm, which occurs in 20% to 25% of patients who are not treated with IGIV within 10 days of onset of fever. Risk factors for coronary artery aneurysms include

- Male sex
- Aged younger than 1 year or older than 8 years
- Fever for more than 10 days
- High neutrophil and band counts
- Low platelet counts
- A hemoglobin concentration less than 10 g/dL
- Fever persisting after treatment with IGIV

Aneurysms usually occur 1 to 4 weeks after onset, but are occasionally seen earlier. Other complications include pericarditis, myocarditis, or endocarditis. The risk of cardiovascular complications makes it imperative that children with Kawasaki disease be evaluated and followed by a pediatric cardiologist.

Keep in Mind

The features of Kawasaki disease may not occur simultaneously. Patients who receive large doses of IGIV should have doses of live, attenuated virus vaccines deferred for 11 months unless there is a high risk for exposure. In that case, vaccinate, but remember to repeat the vaccination at least 11 months after the IGIV is given.

Remember, too, the association between the administration of aspirin to patients with influenza or chickenpox and Reye syndrome. Appropriate measures should be taken to prevent these infections in unvaccinated children taking aspirin.

Part 2

Case Reports in Children Aged 1 to 5 Years

Chapter 12

Fever and a Polymorphous Rash

Presentation

A 14-month-old boy is brought to your office because he developed a fever yesterday and his temperature has not responded to acetaminophen. You saw this child as a newborn at the birthing hospital and he received a birth dose of hepatitis B virus vaccine; you did not see him again until he returned for an upper respiratory infection when he was 4 months old. Your office record indicates that you gave a second dose of hepatitis B virus vaccine and the first doses of DTaP, *Haemophilus influenzae* type b, inactivated poliovirus, and pneumococcal conjugate vaccines and scheduled a visit to get his immunizations caught up.

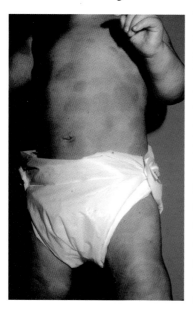

The appointment was not kept and this is the first time you have seen this child in a year. The mother states that he has been healthy and she has not been able to get child care and transportation to bring him for well-child care. The patient lives with his mother, her boyfriend, and 2 siblings who are 2 months and 3 years of age. No one in the family has been ill and the patient does not attend child care. When the mother undresses the child for the examination you are immediately struck by the rash on his trunk and extremities. There are lesions of various sizes and colors. Some of the lesions are red, some are brownish, and some are purple. Most of the lesions are flat, but a few are raised. The lesions are not warm or tender to palpation and do not blanch. You do not recognize a particular pattern to the rash, but it is more extensive on the front of his body (Figure).

You ask the mother when she noticed the rash and what it looked like when it began. She tells you that the patient has had a severe diaper rash for over a week and she thought that the rash on the rest of his body was somehow related. You take off the patient's diaper and find a moderately severe case of *Candida* diaper dermatitis (see Chapter 7). You continue the physical examination. Vital signs taken by your office nurse are as follows: temperature, 39.4°C (102.9°F); respiration, 24 breaths per minute; pulse, 88 beats per minute; and blood pressure, 90/60 mm Hg. The child is well developed and well nourished and in no acute distress. He does not appear to have been bathed recently. Sclerae are clear and tympanic membranes are pink, shiny, and mobile. The oropharynx is normal. Heart sounds are normal, but examination of the lungs is unsatisfactory because the boy has been crying and you hear loud, conducted sounds that preclude hearing crackles or fine wheezing. Neither the liver nor spleen is enlarged, nor do you feel any abdominal masses. His genitalia are normal and both testes have descended. He has a fiery red rash on his scrotum, around his anus, and in the inguinal and gluteal creases. There are red papules and pustules surrounding the areas of inflamed skin. He has good strength and full range of motion of all joints and his neurologic examination is normal with no signs of meningeal irritation. He has a few shotty inguinal and cervical lymph nodes that are not tender.

- **What is your differential diagnosis?**
- **How will you evaluate this patient?**
- **How will you treat this patient's condition?**

Discussion

Diagnosis

Trying to put the fever and rash together you consider *Candida* diaper dermatitis with a hypersensitivity reaction, but the fever would be unusual in this scenario. The variation in size and shape of the skin lesions makes you consider erythema multiforme. You do not see any lesions that look like target lesions and you do not recall this much variation in color; erythema multiforme is usually more uniformly erythematous.

Neither the distribution nor the color of the rash fits with a diagnosis of streptococcal or staphylococcal toxic shock syndrome or scarlet fever. Furthermore, scarlet fever is rare in children younger than 2 years. There are no petechiae and the ankles have few lesions, making meningococcemia unlikely. Even if he did not have this rash you would be concerned; a temperature of greater than 39°C (102.2°F) in an incompletely immunized child makes you consider occult bacteremia or pneumonia. You tell the mother that you need to do some tests at the hospital. You call emergency medical services to take the child directly to the local emergency department. You call ahead and discuss the case with the pediatric emergency medicine doctor.

The emergency medicine doctor obtains a blood specimen for a CBC and differential count and a blood culture. An x-ray film of the chest is also obtained to rule out pneumonia. The WBC is 17,000 cells/μL. The radiologist calls to tell you that the chest x-ray film shows normal lungs and 3 healing rib fractures. You are still concerned about occult bacteremia and elect to give the patient a dose of intramuscular ceftriaxone and hospitalize him. You are even more concerned about child abuse. The 3 fractured ribs are almost diagnostic. Add to that 2 young siblings, a live-in boyfriend, and a child who does not appear well cared for and your index of suspicion rises. At the end of your office hours you go to the hospital and reexamine the patient. The nurse tells you that the mother has gone home to care for her other children. With child abuse in mind, the rash now looks more like multiple bruises in various stages of resolution. You call Child Protective Services to report your concerns and ask social services at the hospital to contact this family. The next day the child is still febrile, but his blood culture is sterile. The mother has talked to Child Protective Services and tells them that the patient often has marks and bruises after she has left him in the care of her boyfriend.

Keep in Mind

Abuse can mimic other illnesses; pediatric caregivers should always have a healthy index of suspicion when the clinical findings do not fit the history.

Conversely, many skin conditions can mimic abuse. These are nicely reviewed in Scales JW, Fleischer AB, Sinal SH, Krowchuk DP. Skin lesions that mimic abuse. *Contemp Pediatr.* 1999;16:137–145.

Chapter 13

Persistent, Painless Finger Nodule

Presentation

It is April and a 4-year-old girl is brought to your office by her father, who is concerned about a sore on the middle finger of his daughter's right hand. The sore began as a red bump near the distal interphalangeal (DIP) joint about 2 weeks ago. The child was well, the lesion was not painful, and the father did not see any evidence of trauma, so he kept an eye on the lesion for the next few days. The bump seemed to be slowly enlarging. The father thought this might be a superficial infection and began to apply an over-the-counter antibacterial ointment 2 to 3 times a day. After a week of topical antibacterial therapy the lesion was not better and perhaps was a bit larger; he decided to have you take a look at the lesion. On examination the child is afebrile and her examination is entirely normal except for a 5-mm, painless, red, papulonodular lesion just below the DIP joint on the middle finger of the right hand. There is no lymphatic streaking or lymphadenopathy. The father cannot recall any scratches, bites, or other trauma to the finger. The family does not have a cat and the father is not aware that the child has played with one. Topical antibacterial therapy has been ineffective; you elect to treat the patient for 10 days with oral cephalexin in case she has a *Staphylococcus aureus* infection.

The patient returns in 2 weeks having taken all of the cephalexin with no improvement. The lesion is now 5 mm by 7 mm and slightly more erythematous. The lesion remains papulonodular without any signs of suppuration. There is still no lymphangitis or lymphadenopathy and the patient remains well except for this lesion. Thinking this may be an infection with a community-acquired methicillin-resistant strain of *Staphylococcus,* you prescribe a 10-day course of trimethoprim-sulfamethoxazole.

The patient returns in 2 weeks with no improvement. The lesion is now crusted in the center and there is lymphatic streaking on the back of her hand (Figure) and the suggestion of a new lesion beginning on the dorsum on her right hand. Careful examination of the right axilla does not reveal lymphadenopathy.

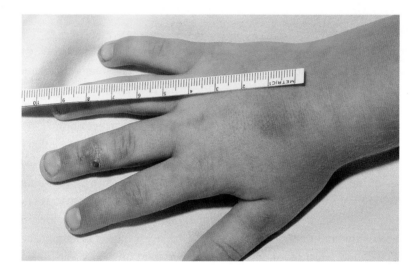

- ■ **What is your differential diagnosis?**
- ■ **Who might you consult?**
- ■ **What diagnostic tests will you order?**
- ■ **How will you treat this patient's infection?**

Discussion

Diagnosis

The non-healing lesion in an otherwise healthy child makes you think about cat scratch disease or sporotrichosis. You wonder what other low-grade pathogens could produce this clinical picture. You ask the pediatric infectious disease specialist to see this patient in consultation. The ID specialist obtains a thorough travel and exposure history. The only travel was a weeklong vacation to Sanibel Island, FL, during the first week of February. The patient spent much of the vacation playing on the beach and collecting seashells.

The father again is unable to recall seeing any evidence of a bite, scratch, or other trauma on the finger. He continues to deny any known exposure to a cat or kitten. The ID specialist confirms the physical examination findings. The differential diagnosis developed by the ID specialist includes cat scratch disease, but this is low on her list because there is no known cat exposure, a scratch was never seen, and the lesion evolved from a painless papulonodular lesion rather than a non-healing scratch with regional lymphadenopathy. The clinical course has been somewhat long for cat scratch disease and the patient has never had signs of systemic illness. The indolent course with the development of lymphangitis and a secondary lesion on the back of the hand suggests infection with *Sporothrix schenckii* or another organism that can begin as a single nodule and develop secondary nodules along the lymphatic drainage of the initial lesion. Infections that can resemble sporotrichosis include blastomycosis, histoplasmosis, chromoblastomycosis, coccidioidomycosis, nocardiosis, tularemia, and atypical mycobacteria infections. Tularemia is unlikely without systemic signs of infection. Sporotrichosis is usually associated with a break in the skin at the sight of infection. A fungal or atypical mycobacteria infection seems more likely. A blood specimen is sent for serologic testing for histoplasmosis, blastomycosis, and coccidioidomycosis and an intradermal tuberculin skin test (TST) is placed with follow-up in 3 days.

After 3 days the TST shows 10 mm of erythema and 5 mm of induration. Results of the serologic tests for fungal infection are pending. The history for possible exposure to tuberculosis is reviewed and is negative. The ID specialist recommends a biopsy for histology, acid-fast stain, and culture for bacteria, fungi, and mycobacteria. You concur and a biopsy is obtained. The acid-fast stain result is negative. Histology shows granulomatous inflammation, but the result of stains for fungi is negative. The reactive TST makes you most suspicious of an atypical mycobacterium infection and the history of a seaside vacation suggests the possibility of infection with *Mycobacterium marinum*. At the suggestion of the ID specialist, you begin empiric treatment with clarithromycin, which has been reported to be effective against this organism in some patients.

Two weeks after the biopsy specimen was obtained the laboratory reports that *M marinum* has been identified. The isolate is sent for antibacterial susceptibility testing.

M marinum, a nontuberculous mycobacterium found in fresh and salt water, causes disease in fish. People can be exposed during leisure water activities or while cleaning fish tanks. Skin infection often follows trauma and exposure to ocean, lake, unchlorinated swimming pool, or fish tank water. The incubation period is usually 2 to 6 weeks. The primary lesion is usually a single, red-to-violet, painless papulonodular lesion on an extremity (eg, finger, hand, elbow, knee, foot). Facial lesions have been reported, but deep infections are rare in immunocompetent hosts. The diagnosis is made by histopathologic examination and culture of a biopsy specimen. An acid-fast stain should be performed, but rarely is the result positive. Histopathology shows nonspecific chronic inflammation and non-caseating granuloma. Langerhans giant cells may be seen. The isolate should be tested for susceptibility to antibacterial agents, but you should keep in mind that susceptibility results do not always correlate with clinical outcome.

Treatment
Superficial infections sometimes will resolve spontaneously or with surgical debridement without antibacterial therapy. Superficial infections also may respond to therapy with a single antibacterial agent. Typically, deep infections require aggressive surgical debridement and combination antibacterial therapy. *M marinum* usually is resistant to isoniazid, aminosalicylic acid,

and streptomycin, but often is susceptible in vitro to a wide range of anti-bacterial agents. Therapy should be chosen on the basis of the results of susceptibility testing. Your patient's isolate was susceptible to clarithromycin, rifampin, tetracycline, and ciprofloxacin. The ID specialist recommended a 3- to 6-month course of clarithromycin. After 3 months of treatment the lesion had completely resolved and the clarithromycin was stopped with no evidence of relapse over the ensuing months.

Keep in Mind
Repeated questioning often reveals a clue that might lead to the correct diagnosis. It is also important to observe the natural progression of an infectious process that is evolving slowly in an otherwise healthy person.

Chapter 14

Vesicles, Pustules, and Crusted Lesions

Presentation

This 4-year-old boy comes to your office because lesions on his face have been spreading and getting worse (Figure 1).

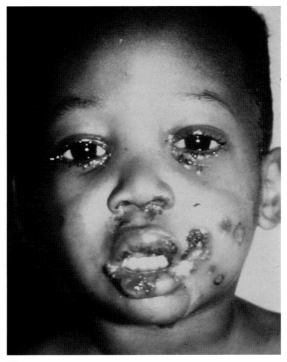

Figure 1

About 2 weeks ago the patient had a cold and developed a sore between his upper lip and nares. The sore was red and had a yellowish discharge that became crusty, and his mother attributed the sore to irritation from his nasal discharge. As the lesion under his nares began to resolve he developed scattered lesions on his arms and legs. When it looked like these lesions were clearing up, new lesions appeared. Over the past 3 days he developed new lesions on his face and around his eyes. The lesions on the patient's lips are making it difficult for him to eat and his mother is concerned about the lesions near his eyes. The mother has also brought her 2-year-old daughter, who began developing similar lesions on her arms about 3 days ago.

The patient is fully immunized and other than the usual childhood illnesses, has been healthy. The cold he had 2 weeks ago was mild and resolved quickly. His sister also had a cold at about the same time. No one else in the family has been ill.

On physical examination the patient appears generally well. He is afebrile and his vital signs are normal. Examination of the skin reveals small vesiculopustular lesions on the eyelids and crusted lesions on the face and extremities. There are areas of hypopigmentation where crusts have been picked off. You also find several enlarged cervical, axillary, and inguinal lymph nodes that are not red or tender. The findings of the remainder of the physical examination are normal.

- **What does this patient have?**

- **Do you want to perform any laboratory tests?**

- **How will you treat this patient's condition?**

Discussion

Diagnosis

The vesiculopustular lesions bring to mind varicella, herpes simplex, enteroviruses, and impetigo. You also consider noninfectious causes such as insect bites and nummular eczema. The fact that this child has been immunized against varicella does not preclude chickenpox. Chickenpox in an immunized child tends to be mild and resolves without complications in less than 1 week. It would be unusual for chickenpox to start as a single lesion under the nares and then continue to develop new lesions over the next 2 weeks. These could represent secondarily infected chickenpox lesions. Primary herpes gingivostomatitis could result in lesions similar to the lesions on this boy's face. The lesions in primary herpes gingivostomatitis usually occur at about the same time and resolve over 10 to 14 days. It would be uncommon to have lesions developing on the extremities and to have new lesions developing over a 2-week period. Enterovirus infections normally occur in the summer and fall and cause vesicular rashes that usually have a single crop of vesicles. The child has not been bitten or stung by insects and has not had eczema or allergic symptoms in the past.

The lesions on the younger sister suggest that this is a contagious disease. The sister has also received varicella-zoster vaccine and only has 2 crusted lesions on her leg. You are relatively certain that your patients have impetigo. The incidence of community-associated methicillin-resistant *Staphylococcus aureus* is high in your region, so you opt to open a couple of the pustular lesions near the eye to obtain a specimen for culture and susceptibility testing to help guide antibacterial therapy.

Treatment

Because of the extent and severity of the lesions on the boy's face, you opt to treat him with oral clindamycin. You prescribe mupirocin ointment for his sister and advise the mother to apply the mupirocin to the girl's skin lesions 3 times a day.

S aureus resistant to methicillin and erythromycin but resulting in a negative D-test are isolated from the lesions near the boy's eye. The negative D-test (see Chapter 25) tells you that the organism is not inducible for clindamycin resistance and you do not need to change the patient's antibacterial therapy.

Keep in Mind

Impetigo still accounts for 1% to 2% of all visits to a pediatrician, 10% of skin problems in children, and 50% to 60% of all skin infections in children. The causes of impetigo have changed over the years. In the 1960s, studies showed that most impetigo was caused by group A β-hemolytic streptococci (GABS) or was a mixed infection of GABS and *S aureus.* The staphylococci were thought to be secondary invaders and patients responded well to antibacterial therapy directed at GABS. Studies from the 1980s showed that approximately 70% of patients with impetigo had a pure growth of *S aureus* from their lesions, while only 1% to 9% had pure growth of GABS. For now, the target organism to treat is *S aureus.* There have also been several studies showing that topical therapy is as effective as systemic antibacterial therapy, which should be reserved for severe cases or patients with multiple lesions on the face.

Keep in mind that skin diseases such as eczema can become infected with *S aureus* (Figure 2).

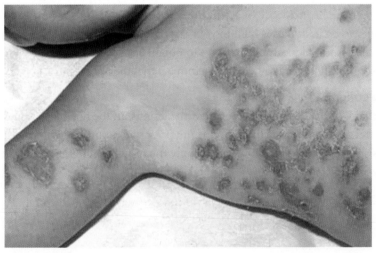

Figure 2. A boy with atopic dermatitis that has become impetiginous.

Chapter 15

Raccoon Bite

Presentation

This curious little boy thought that he would play with the raccoon that was dining in the garbage can behind his house. The raccoon, it seems, was more inclined to dine alone (Figure 1).

The raccoon also broke the skin on the boy's scalp with his claws (Figure 2).

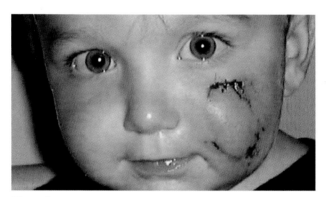

Figure 1

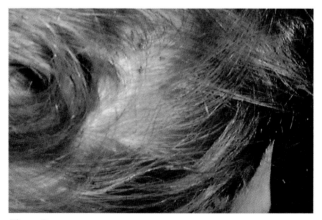

Figure 2

■ **What pathogens are transmitted most often by bite wounds (saliva)?**

Discussion

Diagnosis

For this patient, one of the most important concerns is rabies. Rabies is a common infection in raccoons; this boy will require prophylaxis unless the raccoon was captured and can be tested. You also should determine if the child's tetanus immunizations are up-to-date and give a booster dose if they are not.

Human and animal bite wounds are very common. Dog bites are most common, followed by cats and humans. The rate of infection following bite wounds is highest for cats (approximately 50%), followed by dogs and humans (approximately 15%–20%). The bites of wild animals and exotic pets also can be associated with serious infections, but it is harder to predict what the likely pathogens will be.

The first step in managing a bite wound is thorough cleansing. After sponging away all visible dirt, the wound should be irrigated with a large volume of sterile saline using a 50-mL syringe with an 18-gauge needle. Sedation or local anesthesia may be necessary to clean the wound optimally. Remove any devitalized tissue. Puncture wounds should not be irrigated because the pressure from the saline drives organisms into, rather than out of, the wound. Cultures of the wounds are not helpful unless there are signs of infection. Fist-to-teeth wounds can penetrate the metacarpophalangeal joint; if this is suspected the patient should be evaluated by a hand surgeon.

There is some disagreement about closing bite wounds. Sutures can be a site of infection, so some health care professionals think it is better to approximate the wound edges with adhesive strips or tissue adhesives. Bite wounds on the face are less likely to become infected than wounds on the hands and feet and have greater cosmetic implications. Therefore, facial wounds should be sutured and the patient given an appropriate prophylactic antibacterial agent.

If you are treating a human bite wound you should assess the biter's human immunodeficiency virus status and if the patient is not fully immunized against hepatitis B virus, hepatitis B virus status, as well.

The bacteriology of bite wounds is best known for dogs, cats, and humans. Dog and cat bite wound infections are most likely to become infected with one or more of the following bacteria: *Pasteurella multocida* (or other species), *Staphylococcus aureus*, streptococci, anaerobes, and *Capnocytophaga, Moraxella, Corynebacterium,* or *Neisseria* species. Human bite wound infections involve streptococci, S aureus, Eikenella corrodens, and anaerobes.

Treatment
For minor wounds and scratches, antibacterial treatment is not necessary. Even without any signs of infection, more severe wounds, especially to the hands and face, deserve antibacterial therapy for 2 to 3 days. Oral amoxicillin-clavulanate is the best single drug to treat possible streptococci, staphylococci, *Pasteurella, Eikenella,* and anaerobe infections. *S aureus* infections are not very common following bite wounds, but if signs of infection persist after 2 days of treatment with amoxicillin-clavulanate, consider adding trimethoprim-sulfamethoxazole or clindamycin to treat community-associated methicillin-resistant *S aureus.*

Keep in Mind
If a bite wound becomes infected, obtain a good specimen for culture and let the microbiology laboratory know to look for something unusual.

See Chapter 9 for the management of *Pasteurella multocida* infections.

Chapter 16

Persistent Neck Mass

Presentation

Today a 2-year-old girl is in your office for the third time in recent weeks. She came to your office 2 weeks ago with cervical adenitis. She was afebrile and otherwise well except for the mass in her neck that felt like an enlarged lymph node. There was some erythema of the overlying skin, but minimal tenderness and no warmth to palpation. The mass was not fluctuant. Mouth and throat examination findings were normal. The result of a rapid antigen detection test for group A β-hemolytic streptococci (GABS) was negative, as was her throat culture result. Her past history is unremarkable and no one at home has been ill. Your diagnosis at the first visit was cervical lymphadenitis; you prescribed cephalexin and told the mother that the mass likely would subside over the next several days. A week later she returned, saying the mass in her daughter's neck was unchanged. Thinking that the mass may be caused by methicillin-resistant staphylococci, you change antibacterial therapy to clindamycin. You also consider the possibility of tuberculous adenitis and perform a tuberculin skin test (TST) despite no history of exposure. You check the TST in 3 days; there is some erythema but an induration of only 3 mm (Figure 1).

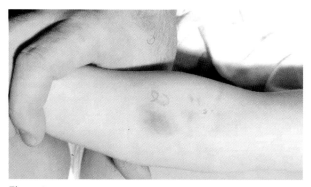

Figure 1

After 1 week of clindamycin treatment, she is back in your office (Figure 2).
The skin over the lymph node is dark red, but there is still no warmth to
touch and she does not seem to be in pain. There is no discharge and
no evidence of a draining sinus. The findings of the remainder of her
examination are normal.

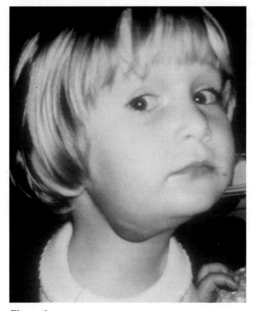

Figure 2

■ **What is your differential diagnosis?**

■ **What other questions will you ask the parents?**

■ **What tests do you consider ordering?**

■ **How will you treat this patient's condition?**

Discussion

Diagnosis

An abscess could persist despite appropriate antibacterial therapy, but the absence of fever and tenderness makes you relatively certain that the lymph node is not infected with GABS or *Staphylococcus aureus.* If the adenitis represented a reactive node secondary to a viral infection, it probably would have resolved by now. A TST with fewer than 10 mm of induration makes infection with *Mycobacterium tuberculosis* unlikely, but the erythema and slight induration makes atypical mycobacteria species a possibility. You also suspect cat scratch disease *(Bartonella henselae),* but the mother denies that the patient has had any exposure to cats. The patient has not been exposed to ticks, raw milk, or wild game, making tularemia or brucellosis unlikely. Other possible diagnoses include mononucleosis, leukemia or lymphoma, actinomycosis, and nocardiosis. The absence of fever makes connective tissue diseases or Kawasaki disease unlikely.

You request a CBC and differential count to evaluate for acute leukemia and to look for atypical lymphocytes that might suggest mononucleosis. You also request a peripheral blood smear to check for lymphoblasts. The CBC and differential count results are normal. The peripheral blood smear reassures you that this is not leukemia, but lymphoma is still a possibility. Epstein-Barr virus serology is negative. The differential diagnosis is narrowing down to atypical mycobacteria infection, actinomycosis, nocardiosis, or lymphoma.

You will need tissue or fluid to make a diagnosis. One of your infectious disease professors used to advocate for needle aspiration, making sure to approach the lymph node through healthy tissue to avoid forming a sinus tract should this be actinomycosis or atypical mycobacteria infection. However, aspiration introduces the possibility of spreading malignant cells that are presently contained. You opt to call a surgical colleague and ask her to perform an excisional biopsy as an outpatient. The surgeon removes the affected lymph node intact and sends it to pathology. The acid-fast stain is positive for mycobacteria. The culture results take 2 to 4 weeks to come back; the isolate from this little girl was *Mycobacterium gastri.*

Treatment

The treatment for atypical mycobacteria lymphadenitis is excision, which is almost always curative.

Keep in Mind

Consider atypical mycobacteria when cervical adenitis does not respond to therapy for streptococcus and staphylococcus. If the TST is positive (≥10 mm of induration) you should start therapy for *M tuberculosis* and continue treatment until you have ruled out tuberculous adenitis.

Although atypical mycobacteria are low-grade pathogens, in healthy children they can cause unusual lesions that do not heal on their own (Figure 3).

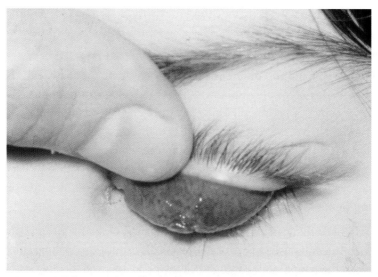

Figure 3. A different child with a bump on her eyelid caused by an atypical mycobacteria infection.

Chapter 17

Red Eyes and Coughing

Presentation

This boy is in your office because his parents are concerned about his eyes, which are very red (Figure). He has had a runny nose for more than a week and now has an intermittent, dry, hacking cough. Despite coughing spells, he has not seemed very ill to his parents. Physical examination findings are normal except for bilateral subconjunctival hemorrhages.

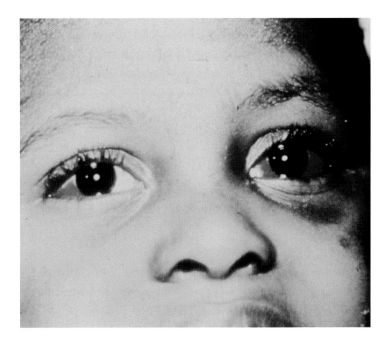

■ **What information would you like from the parents?**

■ **What is the diagnosis?**

■ **What treatment do you recommend?**

Discussion

Diagnosis

The child does not have any signs of conjunctivitis and you are almost certain that the subconjunctival hemorrhage is secondary to the force of his coughing spells. The possibility of a foreign body or reactive airway disease with cough-equivalent wheezing crosses your mind until the patient has a coughing spell in your office. He is sitting quietly when he begins coughing, but once the cough begins he does not stop for nearly a minute and the cough ends with a loud, inspiratory sound. You are pretty sure that he has pertussis. Although he is 4 years old, he has had only 2 doses of DTaP vaccine. His 10-year-old sister has had a cough for nearly 2 weeks, but is not ill otherwise. You obtain a nasopharyngeal swab specimen to culture for *Bordetella pertussis* and ask for a polymerase chain reaction (PCR) test for pertussis as well.

Your clinical diagnosis is pertussis and you plan the management of this patient without waiting for laboratory confirmation. Polymerase chain reaction finding for pertussis is positive, but the culture result remains negative.

Treatment

You explain to the family that it is important to treat the patient to keep the disease from spreading to other people. It is too late for treatment to have any effect on the clinical course of this boy. You also emphasize to the family that everyone in the household is at risk for getting the infection and even if they were not to become very ill, they could spread the infection. They all agree to take erythromycin for 14 days. Azithromycin and clarithromycin are possible alternatives for people who cannot tolerate erythromycin. You also check the immunization status of all of the children in the family and catch them up as appropriate.

This little boy attends preschool. You notify the health department of your diagnosis and give them the family's contact information. The patient and his 10-year-old sister should be kept out of school until they have completed 5 days of erythromycin or other recommended therapy. Children in the preschool who have not been completely immunized against pertussis should receive appropriate catch-up doses.

Keep in Mind

Pertussis is not always easy to recognize after the first year of life, but it remains an important part of the differential diagnosis for persistent cough. Adolescents with recognized pertussis have a paroxysmal cough (72%– 100%), post-tussive vomiting (50%–70%), and whoop (30%–65%); 1% or less will be hospitalized, have pneumonia, fracture a rib, or have a seizure or lose consciousness. Coughing can persist for 3 months or longer. The newly recommended booster dose of acellular pertussis vaccine at 11 to 12 years of age will decrease the exposure of infants to *B pertussis* and the incidence of this disease.

Chapter 18

Fever and Oral Lesions 1

Presentation

In July this child arrives at your urgent care clinic with a fever and sore throat. You see about a half dozen oropharyngeal lesions distributed on the soft palate, pharynx, and tongue. A couple of the lesions are vesicular with surrounding erythema. The remaining lesions are shallow ulcers with a red base (Figure 1).

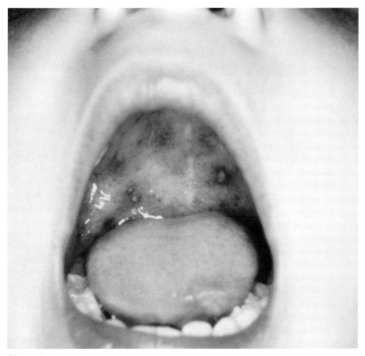

Figure 1

You also find lesions on the hands and feet (figures 2 and 3).

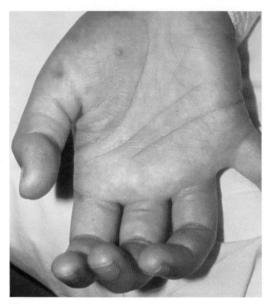

Figure 2

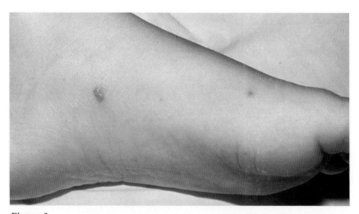

Figure 3

- **What is your diagnosis?**
- **Would you order any diagnostic tests?**

Discussion

Diagnosis

Primary herpes gingivostomatitis lesions generally are located in the anterior portion of the mouth and involve the tongue and buccal mucosa. These lesions look more like herpangina, which is associated with several enterovirus infections. If only skin lesions were present, you would include breakthrough chickenpox in your differential diagnosis. The combination of lesions in the mouth and on the hands and feet during enterovirus season makes hand-foot-and-mouth disease (HFMD) the most likely diagnosis.

The enteroviruses most often associated with HFMD are coxsackie A16 virus (particularly in the United States) and enterovirus 71. There have been a number of epidemics of enterovirus 71 reported around the world, including a major epidemic in Taiwan where central nervous system infection and death was not uncommon. In general, HFMD tends to be a mild, systemic infection characterized by fever and distinctive rash and enanthem. The viruses are spread by oral-fecal or respiratory routes and the incubation period is 3 to 6 days. Virus can be isolated in tissue culture from throat or rectal swab specimens or from stool. In a healthy child, the clinical diagnosis will suffice. Children with immunodeficiencies can become chronically infected and will benefit from identification of the infecting enterovirus by isolation, polymerase chain reaction, or both.

Treatment

In an immunocompetent child the uncomplicated infection is self-limited and does not require treatment. The antiviral agent pleconaril is no longer available from the manufacturer for compassionate use in immunocompromised patients with severe or life-threatening infections.

Keep in Mind

Enteroviruses can be shed by the fecal route for several weeks after infection, and most infections are asymptomatic. Therefore, keeping a child out of child care or school to prevent transmission is unwarranted.

HFMD might better be called HFMBD, with the B standing for buttocks; the rash in Figure 4 is often present in children with HFMD.

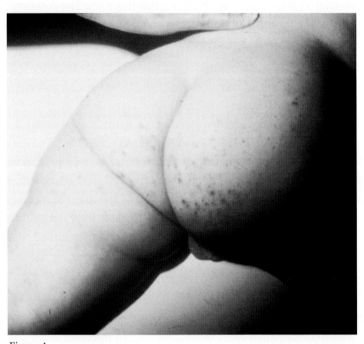

Figure 4

Chapter 19

Fever and Oral Lesions 2

Presentation

This child arrives in your office on a cold January day because she has a high fever and refuses to eat. In addition to lesions around the mouth, she also has vesicles and shallow ulcers on her tongue and buccal mucosa (Figure 1). Her breath smells very bad.

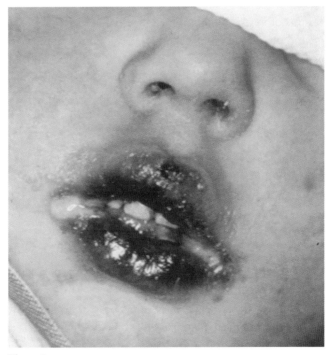

Figure 1

- ■ **What is your diagnosis?**
- ■ **Will you perform any diagnostic tests?**
- ■ **Will you treat?**

Discussion

Diagnosis

Multiple, painful lesions on the gums, buccal mucosa, and tongue of a young child will usually be primary herpetic gingivostomatitis. The oral lesions of herpangina, hand-foot-and-mouth disease (HFMD), and herpetic gingivostomatitis may look alike (shallow ulcers with a red rim), but the lesions of herpangina and HFMD are distributed more on the soft palate and pharynx than in the anterior part of the mouth, as they are with herpetic gingivostomatitis. There are usually more lesions in patients with herpetic gingivostomatitis than in patients with enterovirus infections such as HFMD and herpangina. Aphthous lesions can also look similar, but there are usually fewer lesions and they are more likely found on the buccal mucosa.

Enterovirus infections in temperate climates are unlikely in January. This child has primary herpetic gingivostomatitis. Herpes simplex virus is ubiquitous and you are not likely to identify the source of infection. Most people are infected with herpes simplex virus at some time in their lives. In people with cold sores, most recurrences of shedding are asymptomatic. The most common symptomatic recurrence is the cold sore. You could confirm your diagnosis by swabbing the mouth lesions and sending the swab in transport medium for virus culture. Herpes simplex virus grows quickly and cultures are usually positive in 1 to 3 days. For an immunologically normal child a clinical diagnosis will suffice. If the child has a severe infection or is immunocompromised, you should obtain a specimen for culture by swabbing a lesion and consider treatment.

Treatment

Most children do well without treatment. If the mouth is very sore and the child's breath is malodorous, a mixture of 1 part mild mouthwash, 1 part hydrogen peroxide, and 2 parts warm water can be given to the child to swish and expectorate, or you can gently cleanse the mouth by swabbing with this solution.

Poor oral intake may lead to hospitalization. If children need intravenous fluids it is reasonable to give them intravenous acyclovir as well. Once the child has an adequate oral intake, you can change to oral acyclovir and complete a total of 3 to 5 days of treatment.

Keep in Mind
Secondary lesions can involve the eyes. If you suspect eye involvement consult a pediatric ophthalmologist.

Children who suck their fingers can develop herpetic whitlow (Figure 2).

Note the appearance of primary herpetic gingivostomatitis lesions on the buccal mucosa (Figure 3).

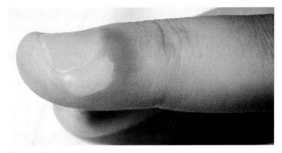

Figure 2

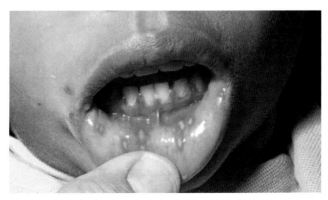

Figure 3

Chapter 20

Bright Red Facial Rash

Presentation

In November, a 2-year-old arrives in your office with a rash. The parents tell you she has had a nasal discharge and some yellow, crusted material in the eyelashes for the past 2 or 3 days. The child has not acted ill and the parents were not worried until the child developed a bright red rash that was most impressive around the mouth, neck, and upper chest (figures 1 and 2). The parents measured the child's temperature before bringing her to your office and it was 38.9°C (102°F).

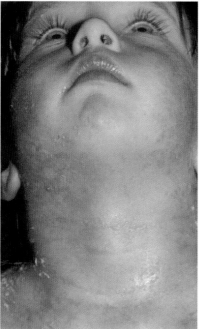

Figure 1

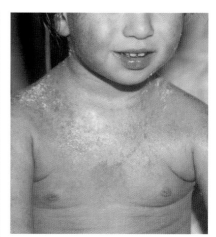

Figure 2

Despite the impressive rash, the girl appears only moderately ill. The
rash extends to the lips, the oral mucosa is normal, and the pharynx
is slightly hyperemic, but there are no petechiae or exudates. There are
bilateral, shotty, tender anterior cervical lymph nodes. The rash is slightly
warm to touch and has a sandpaper texture on the neck and chest; there
is flaking of the skin around the mouth and neck. She says it hurts when
you touch the rash. The Nikolsky sign is absent.

- **What is the differential diagnosis?**

- **What tests would your order?**

- **How will you treat this child's condition?**

- **What will you tell the parents about the prognosis?**

Discussion

Diagnosis

The child has been previously healthy, is fully immunized, and takes no
medications. The parents assure you that she cannot get into the medications in their home and deny any opportunity for the patient to have taken
anyone else's medications. No one in the family has been ill and the parents
are pretty sure that she hasn't been exposed to anyone with a similar illness.
The diffuse erythema of the skin, sandpaper texture of the rash, and hyperemia of the pharynx make you think of scarlet fever. The prominence
of the rash on the face and neck and the tenderness of the rash do not
quite fit with this diagnosis. Conjunctivitis, rash, and red lips make you
consider Kawasaki disease. You also think of toxic epidermal necrolysis
(TEN), but the parents have told you that she has not taken any medications. Stevens-Johnson syndrome could also explain the symptoms, but
there is no involvement of the mucous membranes. Staphylococcal scalded
skin syndrome (SSSS) is the most likely diagnosis. You do a rapid strep test,
which is negative. You send a throat swab for culture.

This little girl has SSSS, which includes 4 clinical diseases caused by staphylococcal exfoliative exotoxin. The extent and type of exfoliation is age dependent. The neonate with SSSS (also called Ritter disease) looks as if she had been dipped in scalding water. The skin is bright red and with the slightest touch, bullae form with extensive skin loss. Non-streptococcal scarlet fever, which the patient here has, and staphylococcal TEN have an abrupt onset with an erythematous rash that has a sunburned appearance, sandpaper texture, and accentuation in skin creases. These symptoms can be indistinguishable from the rash of scarlet fever. Unlike streptococcal scarlet fever, the patient does not have a strawberry tongue or palatal enanthem and cultures are negative for group A β-hemolytic streptococci (GABS). After 1 or 2 days of erythema the patient with staphylococcal scarlet fever will develop cracks in skin creases, particularly around the mouth and eyes. Desquamation of large flakes of skin begins around the mouth and eyes and eventually most of the involved skin desquamates. After 4 to 5 days desquamation is complete, revealing healed skin.

Staphylococcal TEN is initially indistinguishable from staphylococcal scarlet fever, but after 1 to 2 days the upper layers of the epidermis separate, resulting in large, flaccid bullae and a positive Nikolsky sign. Within 48 hours the exfoliated regions dry and desquamate like staphylococcal scarlet fever.

The fourth manifestation of exfoliative exotoxin disease is bullous impetigo. Unlike the other members of the SSSS family, in which toxin is produced at a distant site and carried to the skin in the blood, bullous impetigo occurs when exfoliative exotoxin-producing staphylococci infect the skin and produce toxin locally, resulting in flaccid bullae. An example of bullous impetigo is bullous chickenpox, which is a result of local infection of chickenpox lesions with exfoliative exotoxin-producing staphylococci (see Chapter 24, Figure 6 on page 114).

Laboratory testing should be dictated by the patient's clinical condition. An attempt should be made to isolate *Staphylococcus aureus* from purulent eye or nasal discharge or any other lesion that could be a nidus of infection, and you should document the absence of GABS in the throat.

Treatment

All patients should receive antistaphylococcal antibacterial therapy.
The choice of antibacterial agent should be based on the prevalence of
community-acquired methicillin-resistant *S aureus* and the severity of the
child's illness. Particular attention should be paid to fluid and electrolyte
balance in the neonate with Ritter disease and the child with staphylococcal TEN with extensive exfoliation. Analgesics should be administered
as necessary.

Keep in Mind

Staphylococcal exfoliative exotoxin acts in the epidermis, causing separation between the stratum spinosum and granulosum, unlike drug-induced
TEN, which results in separation between the dermis and epidermis. Thus,
healing of SSSS lesions is usually rapid and without scarring. Treatment of
the staphylococcal infection will prevent further production of exfoliative
exotoxin, but exfoliation continues until the body removes the toxin that
has already formed.

For all but the most severe cases, you can tell the parents to expect a
complete recovery in a relatively short period.

Part 3

Case Reports in Children Aged 6 to 12 Years

Chapter 21

Red Cheeks and Fatigue

Presentation

A 6-year-old girl is brought to your office because of a low-grade fever and a rash that she's had for the past 3 or 4 days. The acute illness is not severe, but she has been losing weight and is disinterested in her usual play activities. When she does play, she tires easily. The parents think these symptoms began about 6 months ago in January of this year, but they are concerned now that the weather is mild and she is not interested in playing outside. When she does go out on a sunny day her face looks like it is sunburned, especially on the cheeks and around the eyes. The redness does not resolve as quickly as sunburn does.

You have cared for this child since birth and she has been healthy except for the usual childhood diseases. She is fully immunized and the family and social history are noncontributory.

On physical examination the patient appears well developed and well nourished, but she is more quiet and less interactive than usual. Her temperature is 38°C (100.4°F), pulse is 82 beats per minute, respiratory rate is 20 breaths per minute, and blood pressure is 96/70 mm Hg. Her face looks slightly flushed and her eyelids are red (Figure 1).

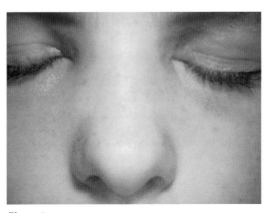

Figure 1

Examination of the skin also reveals pink hyperkeratotic papules over her interphalangeal joints and dry, hypertrophic skin over her knees and elbows. Her eyes, ears, nose, and throat are normal. She does not have lymphadenopathy. Her heart and lungs are normal and you do not feel a mass or organomegaly on examination of her abdomen. Her external genitalia are normal. The findings from her musculoskeletal and neurologic examinations are normal.

- **What is your differential diagnosis?**

- **What else will you do as part of the physical examination?**

- **What laboratory tests will you order?**

- **How will you treat this patient's condition?**

Discussion

Diagnosis

The history of weight loss, decreased activity, and fatigue gives rise to more concern than the fever and rash that brought her to your office. The redness of the eyelids and cheeks exacerbated by exposure to the sun, papules on the fingers, and thickened dry skin on the elbows and knees makes you think that a connective tissue disease is more likely than an infectious process. At this point you remember a part of the physical examination that you do not often perform—examination of the nail-fold capillaries. You recall learning that angiopathy associated with some connective tissue diseases can be seen by examining the nail-fold capillaries. You apply lubricating jelly to several fingers where the fingernail and skin meet. You then set your ophthalmoscope to +40 and focus on the capillaries in the skin immediately adjacent to the fingernail. You are somewhat surprised when you see dilated capillary loops next to areas that appear avascular (Figure 2).

You look in your reprint file and find the picture of a normal nail-fold capillary pattern (Figure 3).

You recall that abnormal capillary patterns in children are most commonly seen in those with dermatomyositis and systemic scleroderma.

The skin findings, weight loss, and easy tiring make you think that the most likely diagnosis for this patient is dermatomyositis. The criteria used to diagnose dermatomyositis include

- Symmetric proximal muscle weakness
- Elevated muscle enzymes (creatine kinase, aspartate aminotransferase, lactate dehydrogenase, or aldolase)
- Electromyographic changes consistent with inflammatory myopathy
- Myositis on muscle biopsy
- Characteristic skin changes

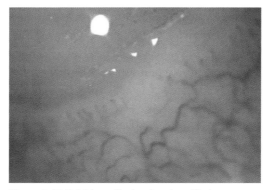

Figure 2. Nail-fold capillaries showing dilation, tortuosity, and dropout. (Courtesy of Robert W. Novak, MD, Children's Hospital Medical Center of Akron, OH.)

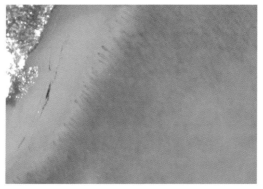

Figure 3. Normal nail-fold capillaries. (Courtesy of Robert W. Novak, MD, Children's Hospital Medical Center of Akron, OH.)

The patient has characteristic skin changes and small vessel disease as evidenced by the nail-fold capillary examination. You tell the parents that their child possibly has dermatomyositis or a similar disease. Because this is not a common disease, you tell the parents that you would like for the patient to be seen by a pediatric rheumatologist for further evaluation and appropriate therapy, if indicated. You call the pediatric rheumatologist to discuss the case, and she makes an appointment to see this patient.

After examining the patient and obtaining the results from the laboratory evaluation, the pediatric rheumatologist calls to relate her findings. On examination, the rheumatologist found symmetric proximal muscle weakness and a markedly elevated creatine kinase concentration. On the basis of these findings and the characteristic skin findings, she is certain that the child has dermatomyositis and should be given systemic corticosteroid therapy. The rheumatologist also adds that she is very impressed that you examined the nail-fold capillaries. She tells you that what you observed is typical for patients with dermatomyositis or systemic scleroderma. You ask the rheumatologist to manage the patient's dermatomyositis.

Keep in Mind

A careful history and physical examination, including some physical diagnostic tricks that we do not often use, can be instrumental in making a diagnosis. Remember that not all interesting cases are caused by an infectious disease.

Figure 4 shows nail-fold capillaries that are dilated and tortuous, but have little dropout.

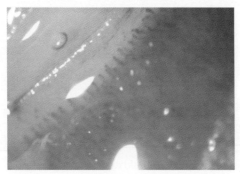

Figure 4 (Courtesy of Robert W. Novak, MD,
Children's Hospital Medical Center of Akron, OH.)

Chapter 22

Fever and Sore Throat

Presentation

A previously healthy 7-year-old girl comes to your office because of abrupt onset of fever, headache, sore throat, and difficulty swallowing. She denies cough or coryza. The other family members are well and the parents are not aware of any sick contacts. School is out for the summer, but your patient attends a daily soccer camp. She is fully immunized and the findings from the past medical history and review of systems are noncontributory.

Physical examination reveals a temperature of 38.4°C (101.1°F), a red pharynx, and moderately enlarged tonsils without exudate. There are petechiae and doughnut-shaped lesions on her soft palate (Figure 1). Her cervical lymph nodes just medial to and slightly below the angle of the jaw are olive-sized and tender to palpation. She does not have a rash. The findings of the remainder of her examination are normal.

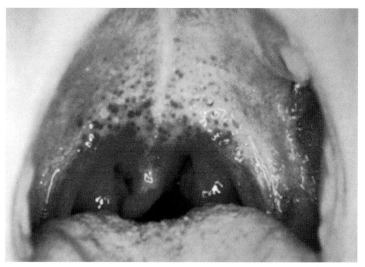

Figure 1

■ **What is your differential diagnosis?**

■ **What diagnostic tests will you order?**

■ **How will you treat this patient?**

Discussion

Diagnosis

Group A β-hemolytic streptococcal (GABS) pharyngitis accounts for 20% to 40% of cases of acute pharyngitis. This means that more than half of patients with fever and sore throat are infected with something other than GABS. About half of patients who have GABS isolated from a throat culture are not at risk for complications or spreading disease and are probably chronic carriers whose sore throat is caused by something else.

A number of viruses can cause pharyngitis. The current season can be helpful in narrowing down candidate causes. In the summer and fall vesicular lesions in the posterior pharynx suggest enterovirus infection. In the winter hoarseness, cough, and fever suggest influenza. In the fall or spring hoarseness, cough, and fever suggest parainfluenza virus infection. Epstein-Barr virus or cytomegalovirus infections are not seasonal, but tender cervical lymph nodes, fever, malaise, and an enlarged liver or spleen might suggest the diagnosis. Fever, sore throat, and conjunctivitis suggest an adenovirus infection.

Group A β-hemolytic streptococci are not the only bacteria that cause pharyngeal erythema, pain on swallowing, and cervical lymphadenopathy. *Mycoplasma pneumoniae* and TWAR (a strain of *Chlamydia pneumoniae)* cause disease, although rarely in children younger than 8 years. These pathogens should be considered in older children and adolescents with cough, hoarseness, and malaise that lasts for more than 3 days (especially in patients with lower respiratory tract findings). A scarlatiniform rash (ie, bright red with numerous pinpoint papules that give the skin a sandpaper texture, and accentuation of redness in the skin folds of the neck, axillae, antecubital fossae, and inguinal and popliteal creases) is highly suggestive of scarlet fever caused by GABS (Figure 2). In patients with a scarlatiniform rash whose throat culture is negative for GABS, consider the possibility of infection with *Arcanobacterium* (formerly *Corynebacterium*) *haemolyticum*. Isolation of *A haemolyticum* requires special media; it is unlikely to be reported from routine throat cultures. *A haemolyticum* is not susceptible to penicillin; the drug of choice is erythromycin.

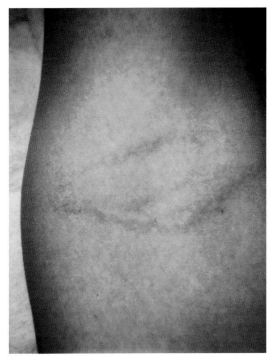

Figure 2

Your patient's symptoms do not suggest any of the non-streptococcal pathogens and you want to test for GABS. You perform a rapid strep test in your office and it is negative. Appreciating the possibility of a false-negative test, you send a throat swab for culture. Uncertain of the diagnosis and knowing that delay in therapy for up to 9 days does not increase the risk of rheumatic fever, you opt not to prescribe antibacterial therapy at this time.

The throat culture is positive for GABS.

Treatment

On the basis of the percentage of patients that remain culture positive for GABS after a 10-day course of penicillin therapy compared with a 10-day course of cephalosporin therapy, it has been argued that cephalosporins might be a better choice than penicillin to treat GABS infections. There is no evidence that the outcome is different after cephalosporin therapy versus penicillin therapy; the American Academy of Pediatrics *Red Book*® continues to recommend penicillin as the drug of choice. Some health care professionals prefer to prescribe amoxicillin because it is more palatable than penicillin.

Keep in Mind

Although GABS continue to be universally susceptible to penicillin, the percentage of isolates resistant to erythromycin is increasing. Consider using a cephalosporin to treat the patient who is allergic to penicillin, keeping in mind that there is some cross-sensitivity between cephalosporins and penicillin.

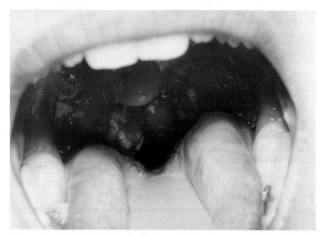

Figure 3. A patient with exudative pharyngitis caused by group A β-hemolytic streptococcus.

Chapter 23

Fever and a Rash

Presentation

It is March and this young man has had a low-grade fever, headache, and malaise for 3 to 4 days. He had been feeling better, but is coming to see you today because of this rash (figures 1 and 2). The rash is most prominent on his cheeks. Close inspection of his arms, legs, and trunk reveal the rash as seen in Figure 2.

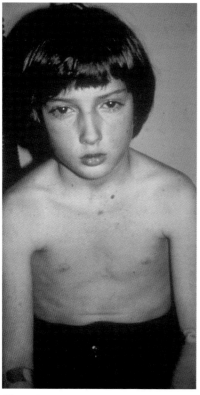

Figure 1

Figure 2

He has received all of the recommended childhood vaccines, but has not
received any recently.

- ■ **What do you see?**

- ■ **What questions do you ask?**

- ■ **What condition does this patient have?**

- ■ **What do you advise the parents?**

Discussion

Diagnosis

The differential diagnosis of the rash includes group A β-hemolytic
streptococcal infections (erysipelas or scarlet fever), roseola infantum,
mononucleosis, toxic shock (streptococcal or staphylococcal), and
enterovirus infections. The bright red rash on the cheeks can look like
erysipelas, but it is not raised, red, and indurated with a well-demarcated
edge, as is found with erysipelas. Erysipelas and scarlet fever are likely to
cause a high temperature, headache, and malaise. The rash does not have
the sandpaper texture on the trunk that you would expect with scarlet fever
and there are no Pastia lines. This child is older than most patients with
roseola and has not had an elevated temperature for several days preceding
the rash. Likewise, the patient has no other signs or symptoms that would
suggest toxic shock syndrome (see Chapter 49). It is March, which makes
enterovirus infection unlikely, even though a wide variety of rashes are
caused by enteroviruses. History and physical findings make erythema
infectiosum (parvovirus B19 infection) the most likely diagnosis.

The appearance of "slapped cheeks" and lacelike rash are diagnostic for
erythema infectiosum or fifth disease. This infection is caused by parvovirus B19. The virus usually is transmitted by respiratory secretions and
symptoms appear after an incubation period of 4 to 14 days. Mild systemic
or upper respiratory symptoms usually precede the rash by about a week.
The rash is often pruritic. The rash can come and go for weeks and is

exacerbated by exercise, bathing, or exposure to sunlight. The diagnosis of erythema infectiosum in an immunocompetent child is clinical. Serologic testing may be more important for immunocompromised patients, patients with sickle cell disease, or pregnant women. A serologic test is available for parvovirus B19, and IgM antibodies remain positive for 2 to 4 months.

Other clinical manifestations of parvovirus B19 infections include polyarthropathy in immunocompetent adults (more common in women), chronic anemia or pure red cell aplasia in immunocompromised hosts, transient aplastic crisis in people with hemolytic anemia (ie, sickle cell anemia), and hydrops fetalis or congenital anemia (first 20 weeks of pregnancy).

Keep in Mind

Parvovirus B19 is ubiquitous and there is not much you can do to ensure that someone will not be exposed. Although infection in a pregnant woman can lead to loss of the pregnancy, only 1.5% of women seroconvert during pregnancy. The risk of spontaneous abortion is about 2% to 4% for a woman infected during the first half of pregnancy. It is not necessary to exclude children with erythema infectiosum from school or child care.

Chapter 24

Suspected Chickenpox

Presentation

A well-appearing child is brought into your office because her mother thinks she has chickenpox. Her temperature is 38°C (100.4°F) and she has about 20 papular lesions scattered on her trunk and thighs. Mother reports that her daughter received the varicella vaccine 3 years ago. The child recently brought a note home from school saying that a classmate had chickenpox. You tell the mother that about 20% of vaccinated children will contract a mild case of chickenpox after exposure and that complications in patients with breakthrough disease are mild. Three days later she returns; you see the same scattered lesions that are almost healed (Figure 1) and a healing lesion on her left thigh that is red, warm to touch, and painful (Figure 2). Her temperature is 38.6°C (101.5°F) and she looks mildly ill.

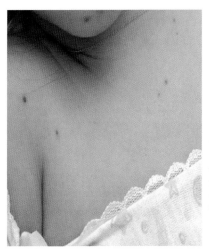

Figure 1

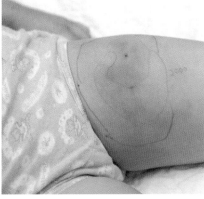

Figure 2

■ **What is your diagnosis?**

■ **How will you treat this patient's illness?**

Discussion

Diagnosis

Chickenpox is changing, but it is not gone. Breakthrough chickenpox generally is limited to fewer than 50 skin lesions and usually resolves quickly without any complications. This little girl developed cellulitis around one of the benign-looking lesions. One of the nastier complications of chickenpox is necrotizing fasciitis. Necrotizing fasciitis starts out looking like cellulitis. Because you don't know whether the cellulitis is going to progress, it is wise to have a surgical consultation in the event that fasciitis develops and surgical debridement is necessary. The pathogen responsible for necrotizing fasciitis is usually *Streptococcus pyogenes* (group A β-hemolytic streptococci [GABS]), but at the cellulitis stage, it is appropriate to provide treatment for *Staphylococcus aureus* as well.

Keep in Mind

Before long, we will not be seeing many cases of chickenpox in unvaccinated children. Remember that uncomplicated chickenpox in an otherwise healthy child can be quite severe (Figure 3).

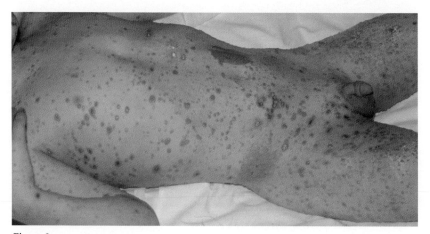

Figure 3

The goal of the current varicella immunization program in the United States is to minimize severe chickenpox, not eradicate chickenpox entirely. Evidence suggests a 2-dose regimen of varicella vaccine for all age groups will decrease the incidence of breakthrough disease. Until eradication occurs, we need to remember the complications of chickenpox.

Additional Cases

This little girl also had chickenpox for 5 days and developed acute swelling of the eyelids. Her temperature was 39.4°C (103°F), her eyes were swollen shut, and the eyelids were very painful to touch (figures 4 and 5). This is GABS necrotizing fasciitis. With debridement and antibacterial therapy, she made a good recovery. After discharge she was seen by an ophthalmologic surgeon to determine whether she would require further surgery.

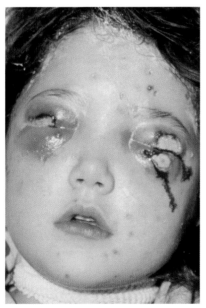
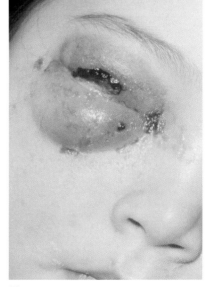

Figure 4   Figure 5

Bullous chickenpox occurs when the chickenpox lesions are secondarily infected with exfoliative exotoxin-producing *S aureus* (Figure 6). Oral cephalexin should be prescribed unless the patient requires parenteral therapy, in which case intravenous cefazolin would be a good choice. If community-associated methicillin-resistant staphylococci are identified from 20% or more of the isolates in your community, clindamycin or trimethoprim-sulfamethoxazole should be used.

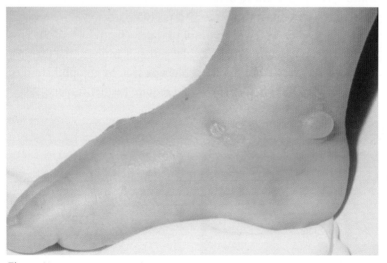

Figure 6

Chapter 25

Persistent Boils

Presentation

This boy arrived at your office 2 days ago with boils on his arm (Figure 1).
You treated him with cephalexin. He is back today and the boils are larger.
The child is healthy and has no underlying conditions or immune system
problems. In the past, you have used cephalexin successfully to treat
hundreds of other patients who had boils.

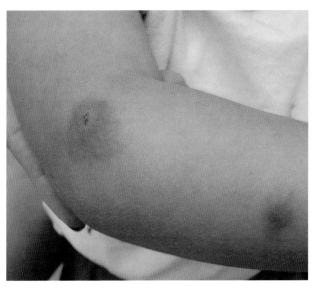

Figure 1

- ■ **Why was the treatment unsuccessful?**

- ■ **What do you do next?**

Discussion

Diagnosis

Boils usually are caused by *Staphylococcus aureus* and sometimes *Streptococcus pyogenes*. It is your opinion that the boil should be drained and cultured.

You refer the child to a pediatric surgeon who requests an infectious disease consultation to recommend an antibacterial agent that might be effective, thus avoiding surgical drainage. The infectious disease specialist is reluctant to treat the patient without obtaining a specimen from the boils because cephalexin failed to cure the boils. The ID specialist also points out that if the boils are caused by methicillin-resistant *S aureus*, drainage is the treatment of choice. The surgeon drains the boil and sends the exudate for Gram stain and culture.

The Gram stain shows gram-positive cocci in clusters that look like *S aureus*. The ID specialist suggests trimethoprim-sulfamethoxazole until susceptibility results are available.

The culture results show the isolate is *S aureus*. Susceptibility testing shows the isolate is resistant to methicillin and erythromycin and susceptible to clindamycin, trimethoprim-sulfamethoxazole, gentamicin, and vancomycin. The D-test was negative. Good guess by the ID specialist!

Treatment

The treatment of community-acquired staphylococcal infections remains a challenge. For a number of years, hospital isolates of *S aureus* have been found to be resistant to multiple antibacterials. It was not until 1999 that healthy children with severe community-associated methicillin-resistant *S aureus* (CA-MRSA) infections were reported.

The resistance gene in community-associated strains of *S aureus* is distinct from the genes responsible for resistance in hospital-acquired strains. Currently, community-associated strains are susceptible to more antibacterial agents than their hospital-associated counterparts, although this, too, is changing. When first studied, only 5% to 10% of CA-MRSA strains were resistant to clindamycin. Now, more than 75% of CA-MRSA isolates from children in Houston, TX, for example, are resistant to clindamycin.

Even when an isolate appears susceptible to clindamycin, it is important for the laboratory to perform a D-test to make sure the strain is not inducible for clindamycin resistance. The test is performed by placing an erythromycin disk next to the clindamycin disk on the culture medium. If the zone of inhibition is flat on the side of the clindamycin disk adjacent to the erythromycin disk (making the zone of inhibition D-shaped), this indicates the isolate may become resistant to clindamycin (Figure 2).

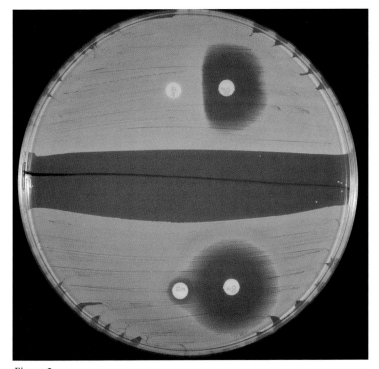

Figure 2

Serious or life-threatening infections that might be caused by *S aureus* should be treated with vancomycin plus a β-lactam (eg, cefazolin). Virtually all staphylococci are susceptible to vancomycin. A β-lactam is included because if the bacteria are susceptible to a β-lactam, it is more active than vancomycin. For moderate and less severe infections, start with clindamycin if most of the isolates in your community are susceptible to clindamycin. Alternatively, you could start with trimethoprim-sulfamethoxazole if group A β-hemolytic streptococcus infection is not a concern.

Keep in Mind
The days of empiric therapy for community-associated staphylococcal infections are rapidly fading. You are wise to keep current on the susceptibility of staphylococci in your community and obtain specimens for culture whenever feasible.

Chapter 26

Bald Spot

Presentation

A 7-year-old boy is brought to your office because his hair has been falling out for the past week and he has developed a bald spot. He has been scratching his head and has had flaking of the scalp that his mother thought was dandruff. The patient is in good health otherwise. The mother has not noticed him pulling his hair, he does not have eczema or another allergic disease, and he has not had a rash or other skin lesions.

Findings from a physical examination are normal except for a bald, scaly, slightly erythematous area on the scalp with thinning hair surrounding the bald area (Figure 1). Some of the hairs are broken off near the scalp and look like dark dots. The remaining hair and scalp appear normal without evidence of dandruff or hair loss.

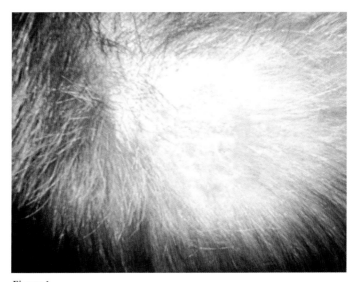

Figure 1

- **What is your diagnosis?**

- **How will you confirm your diagnosis?**

- **How will you treat this patient?**

Discussion

Diagnosis

This looks like tinea capitis (ringworm of the scalp). Seborrheic dermatitis usually involves the entire scalp and generally does not lead to hair loss. Atopic dermatitis generally is not limited to the scalp and is not likely to lead to hair loss. Alopecia areata results in baldness and the bald scalp appears healthy. There is no history of the patient pulling his hair that would suggest trichotillomania. You opt to obtain scrapings to test for dermatophytes and begin treatment with griseofulvin.

With a toothbrush (a scalpel also may be used), you gently scrape scale from the scalp onto a glass slide, add a drop of 10% potassium hydroxide, heat slightly, and look for fungal elements under a light microscope. You see numerous arthroconidia within the hair shaft, suggesting infection with *Trichophyton tonsurans*.

A negative result from a potassium hydroxide preparation does not rule out a dermatophyte infection. Scale also can be inoculated directly onto dermatophyte test medium culture and incubated at room temperature. After 1 to 2 weeks, a phenol red indicator in the agar will turn from yellow to red in the area surrounding a dermatophyte colony. A third option is to send a specimen of scrapings to a microbiology laboratory for culture on Sabouraud dextrose agar. A dry, sterile swab or toothbrush can be used to vigorously rub or brush the area and then replaced in the package to send to the laboratory.

In the past, *Microsporum audouinii* was the most common cause of tinea capitis and could be diagnosed by seeing fluorescence of the scalp lesion when examined using a Wood lamp. Currently, about 90% of cases of tinea capitis are caused by *T tonsurans*, which does not fluoresce, making examination with a Wood lamp of little value.

Treatment

Topical therapy for tinea capitis is not effective. Oral griseofulvin is an effective and well-tolerated systemic antifungal agent that has stood the test of time. Griseofulvin should be given for 4 to 6 weeks. Therapy should continue for 2 weeks after lesions have visually resolved. Oral itraconazole, terbinafine hydrochloride, and fluconazole are also effective for tinea capitis, but have not been licensed by the US Food and Drug Administration for this indication. Shampooing the hair with either 1% or 2.5% selenium sulfide shampoo twice a week until the infection has cleared may decrease the spread of infection.

Keep in Mind

A kerion represents a hypersensitivity reaction to the infecting dermatophyte and often looks like a secondary infection when this is seldom the case (Figure 2). Patients with a kerion often benefit from a 10-day course of oral hydrocortisone with a gradual tapering over the last few days in addition to oral griseofulvin. Antibacterial therapy should not be given unless a secondary bacterial infection can be documented.

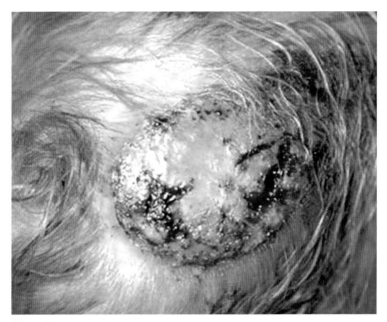

Figure 2

Chapter 27

Fever, Lethargy, and Painful Inguinal Mass

Presentation

Over the past 24 hours this 11-year-old boy has experienced the acute onset of fever, chills, weakness, and headache. In your office, he also complains of groin tenderness and is holding his hip flexed, slightly abducted, and externally rotated. The red and swollen mass in his inguinal region is warm to touch and exquisitely tender (figures 1 and 2). The mass is firm and surrounded by considerable edema. The boy first noticed the mass yesterday and it has been increasing in size rapidly. It has also become increasingly painful. There is no evidence of a wound or infection on the leg. The patient is lethargic, agitated, and appears quite ill.

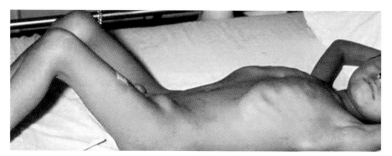

Figure 1

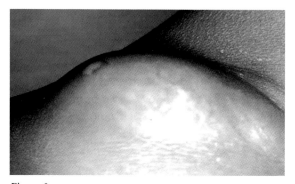

Figure 2

- ■ **Is there any more information you would try to obtain?**

- ■ **What diagnostic tests will you order?**

- ■ **How will you treat this patient?**

Discussion

Diagnosis

On further questioning, the parents tell you that 3 days ago they returned from a week visiting relatives in New Mexico. With more prodding, the mother reveals that most of the trip was spent in Santa Fe, but the day before returning to Ohio was spent exploring the desert. The boy was fascinated by the prairie dogs and had a great time chasing them into their burrows. On further inspection you note insect bites on the legs of the child. The parents admit they, too, have multiple insect bites on their legs. Although the possibility of malignancy crosses your mind, you strongly suspect infection because of the acute onset, intense pain, redness, and warmth. *Streptococcus pyogenes* and *Staphylococcus aureus* head your list because they are the usual culprits. You also consider cat scratch disease, but do not find anything that looks like a slowly healing cat scratch or bite. The boy does not recall any contact with a cat or kittens. The mass is most likely enlarged inguinal lymph nodes, but there is no source of infection in the area as you would expect with streptococcal or staphylococcal infections. Furthermore, the boy's appearance is more toxic than patients with lymphadenitis. Could the boy possibly have bubonic plague?

This young boy is very ill and you want to make a diagnosis and begin therapy quickly. You send him to the hospital for admission and call the infectious disease specialist, asking for input as soon as possible.

By the time you arrive at the hospital, the patient has received a dose of intramuscular streptomycin and has returned from radiology, where a fine needle aspiration of the lymph node was performed. You go to the microbiology laboratory with the resident to look at the Gram stain of the aspirate and talk with the pathologist.

With the help of the pathologist you are able to see the gram-negative rods
with a characteristic bipolar staining pattern (Figure 3). The pathologist is
certain that this is not streptococci, staphylococci, or *Bartonella* and thinks
it might be the first case of *Yersinia pestis* infection he has diagnosed.

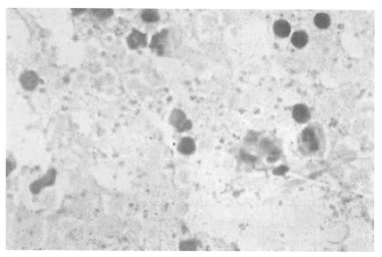

Figure 3

As you walk back to the patient care unit you ask the resident why the
patient was given a dose of streptomycin before the lymph node was aspirated. She tells you that the ID specialist was concerned about the possibility of bubonic plague or tularemia and wanted to start the streptomycin
in case there was leakage of organisms during the aspiration.

Y pestis is transmitted by the bite of fleas from rodents or carnivores.
In the United States, most cases occur in the West and Southwest and are
associated with fleas from prairie dogs, ground and rock squirrels, and
other wild rodents. The incubation period is 2 to 6 days. The usual form
of the disease is bubonic. Patients have fever and large, painful lymph
nodes known as buboes. Inguinal nodes commonly are involved, but axillary or cervical nodes also become infected. Untreated, the patient will
develop chills, headache, and weakness. The mortality rate for untreated
disease is about 50%. Septicemic plague accounts for up to 25% of cases.

In this form of the disease bacteria proliferate in the body and patients become bacteremic and die without developing buboes. A complication of bubonic plague is secondary pneumonia, which has a high mortality rate. Rarely, patients with *Y pestis* pneumonia can transmit the organism by coughing, resulting in primary inhalation pneumonia.

Treatment

Intramuscular streptomycin or intramuscular or intravenous gentamicin should be given for 7 to 10 days or until the patient has been afebrile for a few days, whichever comes later. Because the patient's parents also had "insect bites," they should receive prophylactic oral tetracycline or doxycycline for 7 days.

Keep in Mind

If the history the family provides does not provide clues to the diagnosis, it is important to continue asking questions. Questions about pets, exotic or otherwise, may be helpful. *You must notify public health officials immediately if you suspect a patient has plague.*

Chapter 28

Itchy, Serpiginous Rash

Presentation

This 10-year-old girl comes to your office because she has a rash on her foot that itches terribly and is spreading every day (Figure). She first noticed a red bump between her big toe and second toe about a week ago. Otherwise, she is in perfect health and has been having a great summer on the beach.

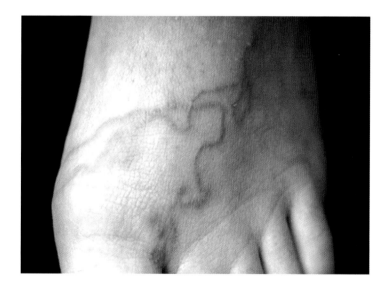

- What is your diagnosis?
- Should she be treated?
- Any recommendations? To whom?

Discussion

Diagnosis

An intensely pruritic, serpiginous track on the skin that advances several millimeters per day is creeping eruption and almost always caused by nematode larvae. Creeping eruption is most commonly seen in the southeastern United States. In this case, dogs or cats allowed to defecate on the beach left behind infective *Ancylostoma braziliense* or *Ancylostoma caninum* larvae. Your patient had the misfortune to get material contaminated with larvae between her toes. A large infestation of *A braziliense* or *A caninum* (rarely other species) can cause Löffler syndrome (pneumonitis). Similarly, if larvae reach the intestine, they can cause eosinophilic enteritis.

The diagnosis can be made clinically. If you obtain a biopsy specimen, the parasite is not usually seen. Instead, you will see an eosinophilic infiltrate. Larvae can be detected in sputum from patients with pneumonitis.

Treatment

Creeping eruption can last for weeks or months, but usually is self-limited. A 10% or 15% aqueous suspension of topical thiabendazole applied 4 times a day for 10 days has been shown to be highly effective for the treatment of early, localized lesions. Treating the parasite is the only way to decrease the intensity and shorten the duration of itching. For the patient with Löffler syndrome, oral albendazole or ivermectin should be considered.

Keep in Mind

Take a comprehensive travel and activity history. Remember that a very pruritic, serpiginous rash on someone who has had contact with sand or soil contaminated by dog or cat feces is likely to be a creeping eruption. Recommend avoiding walking barefoot on tropical beaches, though such advice is likely to be ignored.

Chapter 29

Fever, Rash, and Arthralgia

Presentation

In July, this 9-year-old girl arrives at your office with an oral temperature of 39.3°C (102.7°F), arthralgia, and a maculopapular rash on her hands and feet. She does not have an enanthem (figures 1–4).

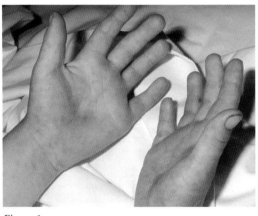

Figure 1

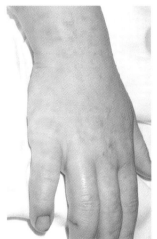

Figure 2

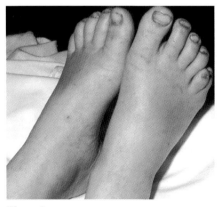

Figure 3

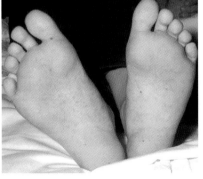

Figure 4

You discover that this family returned from their vacation in rural North Carolina 3 days ago, where they stayed in a rustic cabin in the woods. Seven days ago, their daughter woke up during the night because something had bitten her on the finger (Figure 5). She never saw what bit her and because her finger did not hurt very much, she waited until morning to tell her parents. Her parents were not impressed with the wound and cleaned it with soap and water.

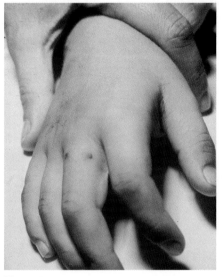

Figure 5

The wound healed quickly and was almost forgotten until she developed her present illness. The girl appears quite ill and you hospitalize her for observation and further evaluation.

- **What is your differential diagnosis?**
- **What further information would you like?**
- **What tests will you order?**
- **Will you begin empiric antibacterial therapy?**

Discussion

Diagnosis

The combination of fever, a macular rash on the hands and feet, and arthralgia could be symptoms of a number of diseases. You are most concerned about Rocky Mountain spotted fever (RMSF) and meningococcemia. You decide to obtain blood for culture and begin administering penicillin and tetracycline intravenously. You have not forgotten about the nighttime bite and can see the well-healed bite marks. What if the biter was a bat? It is too late to inject the bite wound with rabies immunoglobulin, which is best given within 24 hours of exposure. A delay of several days may not compromise effectiveness, but in this patient, a week has passed and the wound is healed. It is not too late to vaccinate. You begin the 5-dose series of rabies vaccine and check to see that her tetanus immunization is up-to-date.

You ask the family about tick exposure and learn that the family was exemplary in their use of DEET. Furthermore, the family wore long pants and long-sleeved shirts while hiking. They went so far as to do daily tick checks on each other and never found any. Your patient is not on any medications and is fully immunized. The patient denies a sore throat or any other prodromal symptoms. You are also wondering if this is the presentation of a connective tissue disease.

The negative tick history makes RMSF less likely, but you send serum for serology. The blood culture should grow *Neisseria meningitidis* if this is meningococcemia. The patient is a bit old for Kawasaki disease and does not have conjunctivitis, mucosal erythema, or the typical rash and has not been febrile for 5 days. Connective tissue diseases like lupus could manifest this way, but you opt to observe her clinical course before pursuing this diagnosis.

In the summer an enteroviral infection is always possible, so you send throat and stool specimens for culture of enteroviruses. Mononucleosis also crosses your mind and you request Epstein-Barr virus (EBV) serology.

You also consider infectious diseases that do not occur often in the United States—tularemia, brucellosis, leptospirosis, and rat-bite fever.

Blood culture results are negative at 24 hours and the patient is dramatically improved. She is afebrile and the rash and arthralgia are almost gone. Epstein-Barr virus serology is negative. You are not sure what you are treating, but it seems to be working, so you continue both antibacterial agents. The patient is doing so well that you send her home on parenteral antibacterial therapy while you wait for outstanding test results. Serologic tests for RMSF, tularemia, brucellosis, and leptospirosis are negative.

The patient has been entirely well since the second day of antibacterial therapy, so you stop the tetracycline and penicillin after 7 days of therapy and the child remains well.

The most likely diagnosis is streptobacillary rat-bite fever. In the United States rat-bite fever is caused by *Streptobacillus moniliformis,* while in Asia the pathogen is usually *Spirillum minus.* Both of these bacteria live in the upper respiratory tract of rodents. *S moniliformis* is transmitted by the bites of rats, squirrels, mice, cats, dogs, and weasels. Laboratory rats can also harbor this pathogen. Haverhill fever is a variation of rat-bite fever that occurs after the ingestion of contaminated milk or water.

The incubation period usually is 1 to 3 days after the bite, but may be as long as 3 weeks. The bite wound heals quickly with minimal regional lymphadenopathy. At onset, the patient has fever, chills, and headache followed by a transient maculopapular or petechial rash that often involves the palms and soles. Approximately half of patients with streptobacillary rat-bite fever have a migratory polyarthritis that is non-suppurative. If not properly treated, the disease tends to relapse.

There are no diagnostic tests.

Treatment

Penicillin G is the drug of choice for rat-bite fever and should be given for 7 to 10 days. Initial intravenous penicillin G therapy for 5 days followed by oral penicillin V has been successful. Alternative drugs include ampicillin, cefuroxime, and cefotaxime sodium. Doxycycline, chloramphenicol, or streptomycin sulfate may be substituted when a patient is allergic to penicillin.

Keep in Mind

The answer is almost always in the history. Pet rats can carry *S moniliformis*. Consider rabies when an animal bites someone and also make sure that the patient's tetanus immunization is current.

Chapter 30

Rash Under a Swimsuit

Presentation

It is Monday morning when this young girl arrives in your office. After a lovely weekend family getaway, this patient woke up with a red, bumpy rash (Figure). The rash is limited to the area covered by her swimsuit and is not pruritic.

She is afebrile and otherwise well. On closer inspection the lesions are discrete, although the erythema surrounding the lesions coalesces in some areas. Some of the lesions have small, central pustules.

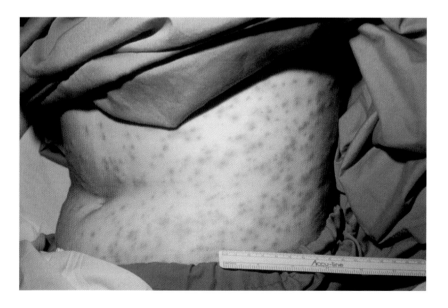

- **What would you like to ask this girl?**

- **What is your diagnosis?**

- **How will you treat this patient's condition?**

Discussion

Diagnosis

The clue is the distribution of the rash; you ask about her activities while wearing her swimsuit. The only time she wore her swimsuit was while relaxing in the motel's hot tub. She does not remember how long she was in the hot tub, but is sure that it was not for more than half an hour. She did stay in her swimsuit and talk to friends for a couple of hours after getting out of the tub. That was Saturday night; she was fine on Sunday and noticed the rash this morning.

This patient has folliculitis and the culture of one of the pustular lesions grows *Pseudomonas aeruginosa*. These bacteria propagate quite nicely in warm water that is not treated appropriately with chemicals to prevent bacterial growth. *P aeruginosa* folliculitis has been associated with hot tubs, whirlpools, spas, and swimming pools. It has also been reported in patients wearing neoprene wet suits and with the use of synthetic or loofah sponges. The skin beneath the swimsuit becomes super-hydrated, creating a friendly environment for *P aeruginosa* to enter hair follicles and proliferate. The skin lesions usually appear within 48 hours of exposure. Healthy people do not develop other signs or symptoms.

Treatment

There is no evidence that antibacterial therapy modifies the course of this infection. The risk of side effects from the use of antibacterials is greater than the risk of allowing the host immune system to overcome the infection. Be sure to let the owner of the hot tub know that she needs to arrange to have the tub disinfected and properly maintained. The rash can persist, sometimes for weeks before resolving.

Keep in Mind

The most important clue to the diagnosis of *P aeruginosa* folliculitis is found in the patient's history. Not every bacterial infection that looks horrible requires antibacterial therapy.

Chapter 31

Fever, Cough, Conjunctivitis, and Rash

Presentation

These children (Figure 1) have just returned from a church-sponsored missionary trip to Africa. Several families from a small, local church spent 2 weeks in a rural African village building a mission school. They returned 1 week ago. Many members of this congregation bring their children to your practice for care because you are tolerant of their religious belief that people should not be vaccinated.

The children developed fever, cough, coryza, and conjunctivitis 4 days ago and the rash you see on their faces 2 days ago. The congregation has met daily to pray for these children.

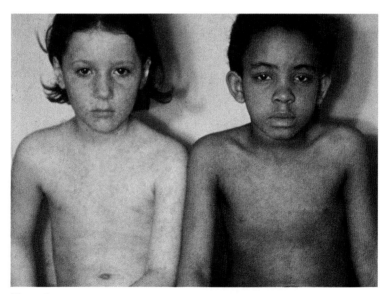

Figure 1

You call the health department and tell them you believe 2 patients have imported measles from Africa. You accept an invitation to go with health officials to examine other congregation members.

Two of the children who went on the mission trip have lesions in their mouths (Figure 2). A third child had clear tears streaming from his eyes (Figure 3). Another child was photophobic and had tearing as well (Figure 4). A fifth child has an impressive rash (Figure 5).

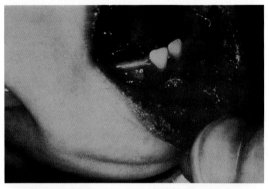

Figure 2

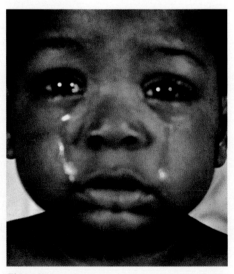

Figure 3

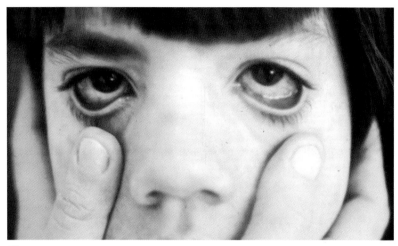

Figure 4

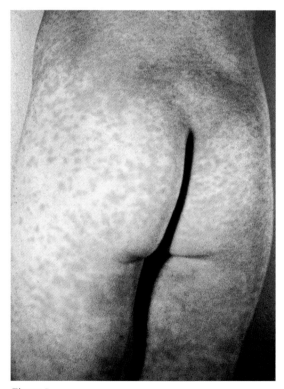

Figure 5

■ **What tests should you order to confirm the diagnosis?**

■ **How do you treat measles infection?**

Discussion

Diagnosis

In the United States, measles is a rare disease. Evidence suggests that we do not have endemic measles, so any case is considered an imported case. If we do not continue to consider measles, we will miss cases and the infected persons will spread the infection. When you suspect a patient has measles, it is important to contact the local health department immediately. Do not wait until you confirm the diagnosis. Preventing spread of the disease is the highest priority. The unimmunized members of this congregation are at risk, as are any susceptible persons they may encounter.

IgM-specific rubeola antibodies become positive early in the disease and remain positive for at least a month. Occasionally the IgM antibody test result will be negative on about the third day of the rash. If you think it is measles and the IgM antibody test result is negative, you should test for rubella and repeat the IgM antibody test for rubeola in a few days. The health department will probably want specimens to send to the Centers for Disease Control and Prevention to isolate the virus for epidemiologic testing.

Treatment

There is no treatment for measles. However, the use of vaccine, vitamin A, and immunoglobulin in selected patients can limit spread and ameliorate disease. Measles vaccine given within 72 hours of exposure can prevent or ameliorate disease. Vitamin A should be given to children 6 months to 2 years of age who require hospitalization for measles.

Children older than 6 months with immunodeficiency, vitamin A deficiency, impaired intestinal absorption, malnutrition, or recent immigration from areas with high measles mortality rates should also receive vitamin A. Consider immunoglobulin for susceptible household contacts, pregnant women, and immunocompromised people exposed to measles.

Keep in Mind

In the United States, measles is a rare disease and a public health emergency. If you suspect measles, call your local health department and let them bring in the troops.

Less-severe complications of measles common in young children include otitis media, bronchopneumonia, laryngotracheobronchitis (croup), and diarrhea. Less-common complications include acute encephalitis (1 per 1,000 cases) and subacute sclerosing panencephalitis, which has been virtually eliminated in the United States by immunization. The mortality rate from measles in the United States is 1 to 3 deaths per 1,000 reported cases.

Chapter 32

Facial Lesions

Presentation

A 10-year-old boy arrives in your office with a rash that appeared suddenly yesterday. The patient is not systemically ill, although the rash is making him quite uncomfortable (figures 1 and 2).

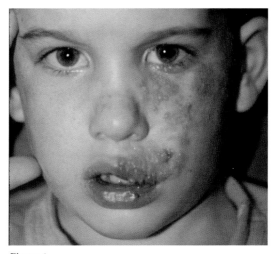

Figure 1

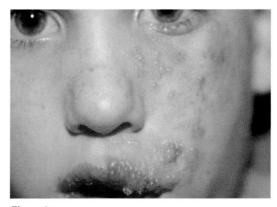

Figure 2

- **What do you see?**

- **What do you think it is?**

- **Would you treat the rash? If so, with what?**

Discussion

Diagnosis

It is summertime and you have seen a couple of children with poison ivy rash of vesicular crusted lesions. Poison ivy rash is usually on exposed areas likely to come in contact with the plant; the vesicles are in a linear pattern. The yellow-crusted lesions on this boy's face could be impetigo, but most of the vesicles contain clear fluid and involvement of the vermilion of the lip is unusual. The vesicular lesions also make you consider a primary herpes simplex virus infection. One of the most striking features about this rash is that it stops in the middle of the lip and is present only on one side of the face. The conjunctivae are clear, but there are vesicles on the lower eyelid. There is no enanthem or rash anywhere else. You ask the mother if her son has had varicella vaccine and learn that he did not receive the vaccine because he had chickenpox when he was 2 years old. On hearing this, you decide to order a fluorescent antibody test for varicella-zoster virus (VZV). You inform the patient that the laboratory technician will need to gently open one of the vesicles and scrape the base to perform the test.

Later in the day the laboratory calls to tell you that the fluorescent antibody test is positive for VZV. You call the family and tell them that the boy has shingles (herpes zoster) and can possibly transmit chickenpox to susceptible individuals. Because they cannot effectively cover the lesions, you advise them to keep the boy home until all of the lesions have dried.

The ophthalmic and maxillary branches of the trigeminal nerve (cranial nerve V) are involved. Your major concern at this time is the possibility of eye involvement. You call the pediatric ophthalmologist and ask him to see the patient today. The ophthalmologist also is concerned about the eye and recommends antiviral therapy. The family fills the prescription and heads home. The next day the family calls because the rash is worse and the lesions on the lips have crusted the boy's mouth shut, making eating and drinking painful (Figure 3). You instruct the family to take the boy to the hospital for admission.

The patient is miserable but afebrile and not systemically ill. You let the ophthalmologist know that the boy is in the hospital and ask him to follow up.

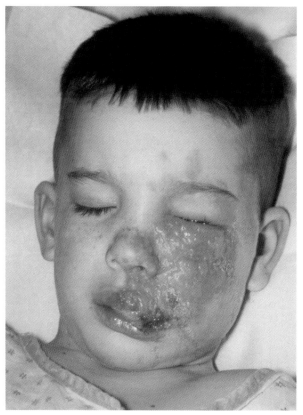

Figure 3

Treatment

In a healthy child, zoster does not usually require treatment. The exception is eye involvement. Most ophthalmologists recommend topical and systemic treatment to prevent or minimize ocular involvement. Systemic acyclovir is the mainstay of therapy in children. Ophthalmologists have the expertise and equipment to properly examine the eye and should be involved in the care of any child with ophthalmic herpes zoster.

In addition to treating this boy for VZV with eye involvement, the kindest thing you can do is gently remove the crusts from his lips and keep them lubricated so that he can drink. Use glycerin swabs to loosen the crusts on his lips until he can open his mouth and then keep the lips moist with glycerin or petroleum jelly.

If clothing covers the lesions, the patient does not need to be kept from school or playmates.

Keep in Mind

Herpes zoster occurs in healthy children and a workup for immunodeficiency usually is not indicated.

Zoster occurs much less frequently in people who have received varicella vaccine than in people who had natural chickenpox. It is likely we will be seeing few cases of zoster in children.

Chapter 33

Snakebite

Presentation

It is a sunny Saturday in July and you are on call for your group practice. At 10:00 am you receive a call from a distraught father who is on his way to the emergency department (ED) at the local hospital. He took his 6-year-old son fishing at a local pond, but the child soon became bored with fishing and wandered over to a rock pile, where he began picking up and throwing stones. The boy screamed and the father ran to find the boy holding his hand in pain. The father caught a glimpse of a copperhead snake darting back into the rock pile.

The father saw a scratch and puncture wounds on the middle finger of his son's right hand. The father immediately carried his son to the car and headed for the hospital. He has called you on his cell phone and asked you to meet them in the ED. You call to alert the physician in the ED to your patient's arrival. As you drive to the hospital you ask yourself the following questions:

- **How do you evaluate the severity of the bite?**

- **How do you treat?**

- **What is the patient's prognosis?**

You arrive at the ED before your patient and talk to the emergency medicine doctor, who has already talked to the poison control center. When your patient arrives it has already been 1 hour since the boy was bitten. He calmed down during the trip to the ED, but clearly is experiencing considerable pain. On physical examination he is slightly tachycardic and his blood pressure is mildly elevated. His capillary refill is 2 seconds. The scratch and fang marks are apparent and already there is considerable swelling of the right middle finger, hand, and forearm. There is no evidence of lymphangitis or pain or swelling of the right axillary lymph nodes. The findings of the remainder of the physical examination are normal.

You carefully measure and record the diameter of the right middle finger and the right forearm and do the same on the left side for comparison. You mark the place where you made the measurements and plan to repeat the measurements every 15 to 30 minutes. You give the boy acetaminophen for pain and send specimens for baseline laboratory studies including a CBC with platelet count, prothrombin time, activated partial thromboplastin time, fibrinogen, electrolytes, blood urea nitrogen, serum creatinine, and urinalysis. While you wait for laboratory results and observe the boy closely for clinical progression, you discuss the case with the ED physician.

Discussion

Venomous snakes in the United States bite approximately 8,000 people each year, and 5 to 6 of those bitten die. There are venomous snakes in all states except Alaska, Maine, and Hawaii. Pit vipers (rattlesnake, copperhead, and cottonmouth) and coral snakes are the only venomous snakes indigenous to the United States. Copperheads account for about 25% of venomous snake bites in the United States; in general, their bites are not considered as toxic as rattlesnake or cottonmouth bites.

Burning pain and progressive edema at the bite site usually begins within 5 minutes of the bite. Edema above and below the bite usually is apparent within 10 to 30 minutes of the bite. Serous or hemorrhagic bullae, lymphangitis, tender regional lymph nodes, or ecchymoses can appear over the bite site 3 to 6 hours following the bite. In a series of patients from West Virginia with copperhead bites, one third of the patients had pain requiring parenteral analgesics, ecchymoses, or swelling of more than half of the bitten extremity; in one third of these patients, the local findings took more than 4 hours to evolve. Systemic signs and symptoms include nausea, vomiting, perioral paresthesia, tingling of the fingers or toes, muscle fasciculation, lethargy, and weakness. More ominous signs are an altered mental status, tachycardia, tachypnea, respiratory distress, and hypotension. Coagulopathy is uncommon with copperhead bites, but occurs frequently following rattlesnake bites.

Acetaminophen did nothing to relieve the severe pain in your patient's finger, so you start to give intravenous morphine. During the next 3 hours, the local findings progress. His hand and forearm continue to swell, he develops lymphangitis, and a large hemorrhagic bullous lesion appears at the site of the bite (Figure). The pain management allows the patient's heart rate and blood pressure to normalize and he has no other signs or symptoms of systemic disease. All of his baseline laboratory results are normal. Because of the progression of his local findings, you hospitalize the patient and ask the hand surgeon to provide consultation in case there is a need to decompress the hand to protect function.

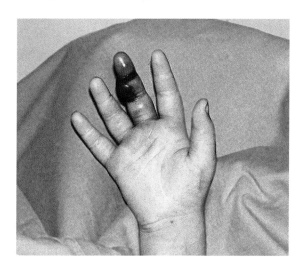

Treatment

First aid measures such as the use of tourniquets, incision and suction, and the application of ice, which have been recommended in the past, are now discouraged. You should always contact a regional poison center to help you guide the management of a patient bitten by a native or exotic snake. Indications for use of antivenin after a rattlesnake bite include worsening local injury, coagulopathy, or systemic effects such as hypotension or an altered mental status. Indications for the use of antivenin are not defined clearly for copperhead bites. A recent study of copperhead bites suggests that antivenin therapy should be considered if the patient requires parenteral analgesia, ecchymosis is present, or there is swelling of more than half of the involved extremity. On the basis of these recommendations, you consider antivenin therapy for your patient and call the poison control center and the manufacturer for their treatment recommendations.

Your patient was infused with 6 vials of Crotalidae Polyvalent Immune Fab (ovine) antivenin (CroFab, Savage Laboratories, Melville, NY), with an additional 2 vials given at 6, 12, and 18 hours. He had no further progression of local symptoms after the initial infusion of antivenin and improved quickly over the next 3 days. The bullous lesion resolved without surgical intervention.

Keep in Mind

If you do not have the number of your regional poison control center, call the national hotline at 800/222-1222 to be connected with your regional center.

Chapter 34

Swelling Behind the Ear

Presentation

A 6-year-old boy was in your office 3 days ago with an acute onset of fever and left ear pain. On physical examination he had a red, bulging tympanic membrane with an obvious air fluid level. He has had several episodes of acute otitis media in the past and you have discussed the possibility of placement of pressure equalization tubes with his parents. You prescribed high-dose amoxicillin.

He is in your office today because he still has fever (oral temperature of 38.4°C [101.1°F]) and ear pain and now his left ear is sticking out; he has redness and a painful swelling behind this ear (figures 1 and 2).

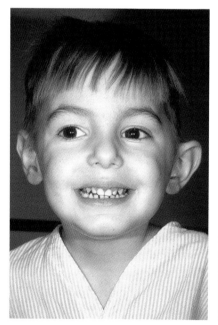 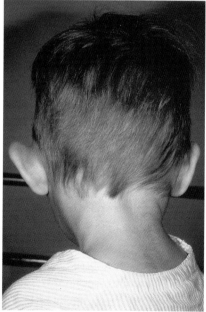

Figure 1   Figure 2

On physical examination you note that the red, tender, and fluctuant swelling behind the left ear displaces the auricle of the ear inferiorly and anteriorly. The left tympanic membrane is perforated and there is pus in the external auditory canal. The findings of the remainder of the examination are normal.

- **What is your diagnosis?**

- **What further evaluation is indicated?**

- **How should this child's infection be treated?**

Discussion

Diagnosis

This child has mastoiditis. The extent of disease must now be ascertained to determine the appropriate therapeutic interventions.

The infection can spread to the periosteum without bone involvement or can involve the bone and may result in a subperiosteal abscess. The fluctuance of the postauricular swelling makes you suspect that your patient has a subperiosteal abscess. Further spread of infection can involve the petrous portion of the temporal bone or rarely may involve the neck muscles that attach to the tip of the mastoid. Involvement of the petrous portion of the temporal bone can result in ipsilateral eye pain and paralysis of the external rectus muscle. Computed tomography of the temporal bone should be performed to determine the extent of disease; an otolaryngologist should be consulted.

In a recent study of 86 children with mastoiditis, children older than 2 years had higher rates of previous otologic problems, earache, and purulent discharge (about one third of the patients were younger than 2 years). The bacteria most commonly isolated from the children younger than 2 years were *Streptococcus pneumoniae,* while *Pseudomonas aeruginosa* were the bacteria most commonly isolated in the group of older children. The investigators questioned whether *P aeruginosa* was the pathogen or represented contamination from the external auditory canal. Most patients with *P aeruginosa* isolates recovered without giving anti-pseudomonal antibacterial agents, supporting the idea that these isolates usually represent contamination.

Treatment

All children with mastoiditis require parenteral antibacterial therapy. It is best to wait until an optimal specimen to culture for bacterial pathogens has been obtained before beginning antibacterial therapy. If computed tomography does not show bony involvement, the infection can be treated by performing a myringotomy and prescribing parenteral antibacterial therapy. If there is involvement of the temporal bone the child will require a mastoidectomy. The extent of surgery will depend on the disease process. This patient had a subperiosteal abscess that was drained. Initial antibacterial therapy with ceftriaxone should cover the usual pathogens associated with acute otitis media. It may be necessary to change antibacterial agents based on susceptibility testing of isolates from the middle ear or mastoid.

Keep in Mind

Technically, all cases of acute otitis media involve the mastoid air cells because the middle ear and the mastoids are in direct communication. With effective antibacterial therapy, inflammation of the mastoid air cells resolves along with the otitis.

Mastoiditis was much more common in the pre-antibacterial era, but remains a potential complication of otitis media. The incidence of mastoiditis has not increased as pneumococcal resistance to antibacterial agents has increased, although this remains a possibility.

Chapter 35

Fever, Rash, and Vomiting

Presentation

A 9-year-old boy arrives in your office in early December with a 3-day history of fever, headache, sore throat, and rash that began yesterday and is much more extensive today. He vomited twice last night and has been tired and achy for the past 2 days. The patient is well-known to you; he has been fully immunized and has never been seriously ill. No one in his family is ill and there are no known sick contacts. The rash started on his face and neck and has spread to his trunk and extremities.

On physical examination the patient appears ill and has an obvious, bright red rash and circumoral pallor (Figure 1). His temperature is 39.4°C (102.9°F), pulse is 80 beats per minute, respiratory rate is 18 breaths per minute, and blood pressure is 104/72 mm Hg.

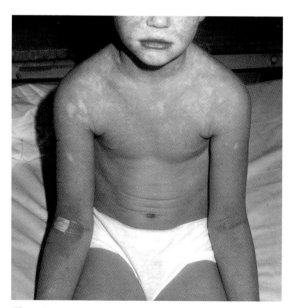

Figure 1

His skin is bright red with numerous pinpoint papules that give his skin a sandpaper texture. The skin does not seem to be painful when you touch it. There is accentuation of redness in the skin folds of his neck, axillae, antecubital fossae, and inguinal and popliteal creases. The rash is not as uniform on his face, but the redness of the rash and his cherry red lips give the impression of circumoral pallor. The rash has not involved his palms or soles. His conjunctivae are clear, ears are normal, tongue has a yellowish-white coating with protruding red papillae, and pharynx is red with 3+ enlarged tonsils without exudate. You also note petechiae and doughnut-shaped lesions on his hard and soft palate. His lungs are clear to auscultation and cardiovascular examination is normal. His abdomen is soft without mass or organomegaly. Musculoskeletal and neurologic examinations are normal.

- ■ **What is your differential diagnosis?**
- ■ **What additional information would you like from the parents?**
- ■ **What laboratory tests would you obtain?**
- ■ **How will you manage this patient's condition?**

Discussion

Diagnosis

This patient's symptoms are not something you see every day. You are worried about staphylococcal or streptococcal toxic shock syndrome. You also are considering the possibility of scarlet fever or staphylococcal scarlatina. Kawasaki disease is another possibility, but 80% of patients with Kawasaki disease are younger than 5 years. He also does not have conjunctivitis or involvement of his hands and feet. You consider measles, as well. However, he has had 2 doses of MMR vaccine, there has not been a case of measles in your community for years, and he has not traveled or been exposed to anyone who has been out of the country. His high fever, headache, sore throat, and signs of systemic illness make staphylococcal scarlatina unlikely. You also consider mononucleosis, but an extensive rash in a patient who has not received antibacterial therapy (which he has not) makes this diagnosis unlikely. The parents have not given the child any medications and to their knowledge there is nothing he could have taken. The patient also denies having taken any medications. Thus, a drug reaction is unlikely. The normal blood pressure makes toxic shock less likely, but you are still concerned enough to hospitalize the child for evaluation, observation, and antibacterial therapy.

A rapid test for group A β-hemolytic streptococci (GABS) is positive. You send a throat culture to confirm this result. You are nonetheless concerned that this patient could have early staphylococcal toxic shock syndrome. You obtain appropriate laboratory tests to evaluate renal and hepatic function, a CBC and differential count (paying particular attention to the platelet count), and a creatinine phosphokinase concentration and check for disseminated intravascular coagulation (see Chapter 37). You also send a blood specimen to culture for bacteria. Although you are considering scarlet fever, you want to provide treatment for *Staphylococcus aureus* infection as well as GABS, so you begin therapy with vancomycin and clindamycin. You ask the on-call pediatric intensivist to consult so that everyone is prepared in the event the boy deteriorates.

The WBC count is 15,000 cells/μL and platelet count is normal, as are electrolytes, creatinine, blood urea nitrogen, and liver function tests. There is no evidence of intravascular coagulation. The next day the patient feels somewhat better. His blood culture result is negative and his throat culture is growing GABS. You change his antibacterial therapy to oral penicillin V and discharge the patient home.

You see him in your office for follow-up 2 days later. He is afebrile and there is some desquamation on his face and trunk (Figure 2).

His tongue now has the typical red strawberry appearance (Figure 3).

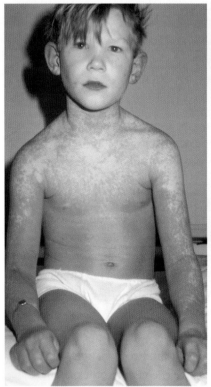

Figure 2

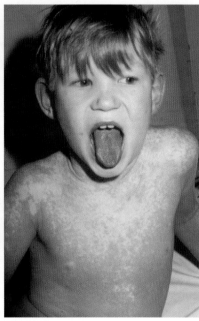

Figure 3

Treatment
The treatment for scarlet fever is the same as for GABS pharyngitis— 10 days of oral penicillin.

Keep in Mind
Scarlet fever is GABS pharyngitis caused by a strain of streptococcus that produces pyrogenic exotoxin. Scarlet fever also can occur with skin and soft tissue infections such as surgical wound infections, giving rise to

surgical scarlet fever. Antibodies against the pyrogenic exotoxin protect against toxin-mediated aspects of the disease, but not against subsequent GABS infections. By the age of 10 years about 80% of children have protective antibodies, explaining why scarlet fever is most often seen in children 4 to 8 years old.

It is important to advise parents about what they should expect as their child convalesces. The rash fades over 5 to 7 days and is followed by peeling that usually begins on the face and trunk. Peeling is most extensive on the hands and feet and in the axillae and groin. Desquamation may continue for weeks. After weeks to months, transverse lines on the fingernails and toenails (Beau lines) may become apparent. Some children will experience temporary hair loss.

If not treated properly, children with scarlet fever are at risk for rheumatic fever.

Chapter 36

Fever, Rash, and Facial Nerve Palsy

Presentation

It is August and every day several children with fever and rash (mostly caused by enteroviral infection) arrive in your office. A 6-year-old boy arrives with fever, headache, a stiff neck, and a rash (Figure 1).

A close inspection of the rash reveals more detail (Figure 2).

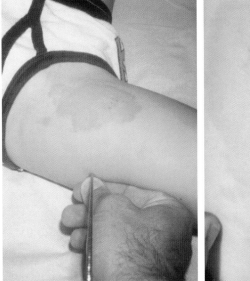 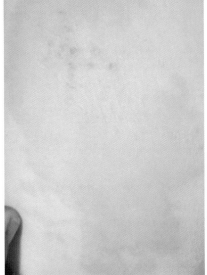

Figure 1   Figure 2

You discover that the family vacationed in New Hampshire the first weekend in July, and they had a great time camping and hiking. No one in the family was ill on the trip or subsequently. Their little boy was fine until about a week ago when he developed a fever and a rash on his inner thigh. Two days ago he complained of a headache and later, a sore neck. The family decided to see you today when they noticed that the left side of the boy's mouth was not moving when he spoke and his speech was slurred. His left eyebrow sagged and he could not close his left eye all the way.

The boy is ill, but does not have a toxic appearance. His oral temperature is 39.6°C (103.3°F). He has a positive Brudzinski sign and right facial nerve palsy, but does not have papilledema. Except for the rash, the findings of the remainder of his examination are normal.

- **What is your differential diagnosis?**
- **What other information would you obtain from the parents?**
- **What, if any, diagnostic tests do you order?**
- **Is this something you can treat, and if so, with what?**

Discussion

Diagnosis

The parents do not recall finding any ticks on the child while in New Hampshire, but none of the family members used insect repellent before hiking even though they were wearing shorts and T-shirts most of the time. You have seen a wide variety of enteroviral rashes this summer, but this rash resembles erythema migrans and you wonder if this could be Lyme disease. You are also concerned that this child may have meningitis and consider meningococcal disease, even though the rash is not petechial or purpuric.

You send the family to the local emergency department (ED), where it will be easier to obtain blood for a CBC count and perform a lumbar puncture. The WBC count is 12,000 cells/μL with a predominance of lymphocytes and mononuclear cells. The cerebrospinal fluid (CSF) has 73 WBCs and they are all mononuclear cells. The protein is 76 mg/dL and glucose is 50 mg/dL. The finding from the Gram stain of the CSF is negative. You request a polymerase chain reaction test of CSF for enteroviruses. You send blood for culture and admit the boy to the hospital.

This child has early disseminated Lyme disease with meningitis and seventh nerve palsy. Ticks transmit Lyme disease caused by *Borrelia burgdorferi* during feeding. On the East Coast and in the upper Midwest of the United States, the tick vector is *Ixodes scapularis;* on the West Coast, the vector is *Ixodes pacificus.* The incubation from time of tick bite to the appearance of erythema migrans typically is 7 to 14 days, but can range from 3 to 31 days.

Enteroviral meningitis and Lyme meningitis follow different clinical courses. Patients with enteroviral meningitis are usually seen a day or 2 after onset, while patients with Lyme meningitis have symptoms for 4 to 17 days before seeing a health care professional. Most patients with Lyme or enteroviral meningitis will have neck symptoms. Children with Lyme meningitis will usually have had a headache for several days, compared with 1 day for patients with enteroviral meningitis. The most important symptom in this boy is his seventh nerve palsy. Cranial neuropathy, most commonly seventh nerve palsy, occurs in more than half of children with Lyme meningitis and is very rare in patients with enteroviral meningitis. The majority of children with enteroviral meningitis are younger than 1 year, while Lyme meningitis usually occurs in children older than 4 years. Meningococcal meningitis usually has an acute onset and the CSF and peripheral blood have a predominance of polymorphonuclear neutrophils.

Clinical manifestations of Lyme disease are divided into early localized, early disseminated, and late. The goal of the clinician is to recognize and treat early disease, thereby preventing late disease. Erythema migrans is the most distinctive feature of early disease. A red macule or papule expands over days or weeks into a large, annular, erythematous lesion that often shows central clearing. Vesicles may be present (Figure 2). Common systemic symptoms include fever, malaise, joint or muscle pain, headache, and neck stiffness.

Early disseminated disease most commonly manifests as multiple areas of erythema migrans 3 to 5 weeks after the tick bite. Lesions, though smaller, appear similar to the primary lesion. Systemic symptoms are similar to those seen in early, localized disease, but also include cranial nerve palsies (especially seventh), meningitis, and conjunctivitis.

Late disease is uncommon in children treated for early disease. When it does occur it usually manifests as large-joint pauciarticular arthritis, most commonly in the knees. Central nervous system involvement in late disease is rare in children.

The diagnosis of early disease is based on clinical manifestations. Serologic test results do not become positive until 3 to 6 weeks have passed and may not become positive at all in patients who are treated early. Once positive, Lyme antibodies persist for years and must be interpreted with care. Enzyme immunoassay performed in a reference laboratory is the best test for detecting antibody and should be confirmed by a Western immunoblot.

Treatment
For children younger than 8 years amoxicillin is given for 14 to 21 days. Doxycycline should be used for children 8 years and older. Patients with meningitis should receive ceftriaxone. Prophylactic antibacterial therapy following a tick bite is not recommended.

Keep in Mind
To remove a tick, grasp it with fine tweezers as close to the skin as possible and gently pull it straight out—no twisting. If tweezers are not available fingers will do, but protect them with tissue and wash your hands immediately.

Chapter 37

Fever and a Petechial Rash

Presentation

On a sunny day in mid-August, this 11-year-old boy is in your office because of a fever of 40°C (104°F) and an erythematous, macular, petechial rash (Figure 1). The findings of the rest of the physical examination are benign.

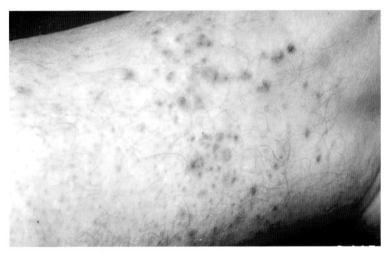

Figure 1

The family is from South Carolina and is in town to visit relatives. They have been away from home for nearly 1 week. The boy was well until last night when he developed fever. The family was not concerned until this morning when they noticed the rash. The parents know about Rocky Mountain spotted fever (RMSF) and make sure you know that they inspect for, find, and remove ticks on a regular basis. They are sure he had ticks on him in the days preceding his trip. There are 2 other children in the family, but both are well.

- **What possible diagnoses are you thinking about?**

- **What information do you want?**

- **What do you do next?**

Discussion

Diagnosis

Your chief concerns at this time are RMSF and meningococcemia. A fair number of local children have been seen with fever, a petechial rash, and meningitis associated with echovirus 9 infections. The possibility of Henoch-Schönlein purpura also exists, but you keep that diagnosis low on your list because it is not often associated with a high fever. You do not take any chances and send the family to the emergency department (ED) for further evaluation and treatment.

You call ahead to the ED and let them know that you are worried about this child and want him to be evaluated for sepsis and treated for meningo-coccemia and RMSF as quickly as possible. When the boy arrives in the ED his temperature is still 40°C (104°F), his blood pressure is normal for age, he is tachycardic, and his respiratory rate is normal. The child still appears normal and is interactive. Blood is obtained for a CBC and differential count, a metabolic screen, diffuse intravascular coagulation panel (prothrombin time, partial thromboplastin time, D dimers, and fibrinogen), and culture. An intravenous line is placed and ceftriaxone, vancomycin, and doxycycline are ordered by the ED physician. A lumbar puncture is performed. The boy is admitted to the pediatric intensive care unit in case his condition deteriorates.

In addition to the history obtained in your office, the admitting resident learns that the patient has received 4 doses of Hib conjugate vaccine. He did not receive pneumococcal conjugate vaccine because he was too old when it reached the market.

The laboratory results show a total WBC count of 2,500 cells/μL with a left shift. The CSF has 2 WBCs, no RBCs, and normal protein and glucose. There is no evidence of disseminated intravascular coagulation. By the time you arrive at the hospital, the patient appears as depicted in Figure 2.

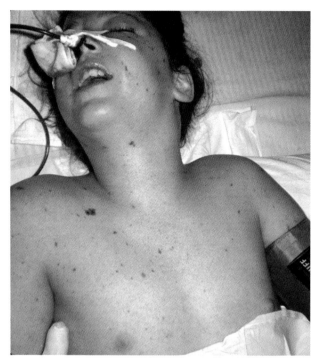

Figure 2

The clinical diagnosis is meningococcemia. You call the local health department to report the presumptive diagnosis. The antibacterials given in the ED were ceftriaxone, vancomycin, and doxycycline. The child is more tachycardic and the intensivist has begun fluid therapy to treat shock. After about 14 hours of incubation the blood culture is growing gram-negative diplococci in pairs. Vancomycin and doxycycline are stopped. The patient stabilizes with bolus fluid therapy and does not require pressors. A repeat CBC the day after hospitalization reveals 12,000 WBCs/μL and is shifted far to the left. You are worried about the blood supply to some of the purpuric lesions and ask a plastic surgeon to consult. You thank the intensivist for outstanding anticipatory management.

Treatment

Although penicillin is still very effective for the treatment of *Neisseria meningitidis* in most countries, ceftriaxone, cefotaxime, and ampicillin are equally effective. Seven days of antimicrobial therapy is adequate.

An important part of the management of meningococcal disease is identifying high-risk contacts and giving antibacterial prophylaxis as soon as possible after the diagnosis is made. Rifampin twice a day for 2 days, a single dose of intramuscular ceftriaxone, or for adults, a single oral dose of ciprofloxacin are equally effective in eradicating *N meningitidis* from the pharynx. High-risk contacts include household contacts during the 7 days before the onset of illness, child care or nursery school contacts, persons directly exposed to the patient's secretions, persons performing mouth-to-mouth resuscitation, or those in contact with respiratory secretions during intubation.

Keep in Mind

Respect and fear *N meningitidis*. Fulminant meningococcemia can be fatal in hours despite optimal antibacterial and supportive therapy. Always take a petechial rash seriously.

Patients with C3, C5–C9, or properdin deficiencies or asplenia (anatomic or functional) are at increased risk of infection and recurrence.

Complications of meningococcemia such as arthritis and pericarditis can present when you think the patient is well along the road to recovery.

Chapter 38

Extremity Rash and Pruritus

Presentation

An 11-year-old, active, healthy boy, well-known to you, arrives in your office. His previous visits, other than well-child care, were for sutures, sprains, a nail puncture wound, and a broken arm. Now he is in your office with a rash and pruritus (Figure). The rash appeared today, but he recalls being itchy a few days ago.

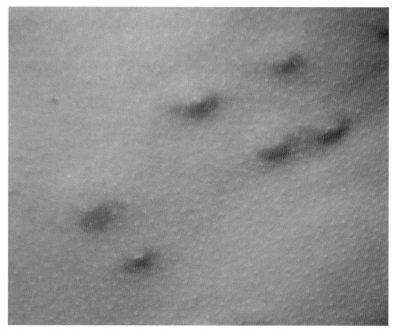

Figure 1 (Douglas Hoffman, MD, Dermatlas; www.dermatlas.org. Reprinted with permission.)

- ■ **What is your differential diagnosis?**

- ■ **What are you going to ask this boy and his parents?**

- ■ **How do you treat this patient's condition?**

Discussion

Diagnosis

The rash appears to be urticaria and pruritus is his major complaint; what could be the cause? He has never had an allergic reaction to anything in the past. He does not have eczema or asthma, nor does anyone in the family. You ask him and his father about new foods, clothes, laundry detergent, soaps, sun protection, insect repellent, or anything else they can think of that could have resulted in contact or systemic allergy. They do not recall anything new or different in his routine that could provide a novel exposure.

The rash is only on his legs, so you can rule out a systemic cause. You consider reactions to plants, but it does not look like the rashes caused by poison ivy, oak, or sumac. With much coaxing, your patient confesses to wading in a "strictly off-limits" neighborhood pond to retrieve a ball. It was not too long after this that his legs started itching. The itching subsided and he forgot about his little adventure until the rash broke out today.

You consider swimmer's itch (although he was not exactly swimming). Swimmer's itch is also called cercarial or schistosome dermatitis. This aggravating condition is caused by avian and nonhuman mammalian species of *Schistosoma*. *Schistosoma* eggs are excreted by the host (mammalian or avian) into fresh water, where they hatch into motile miracidia. The miracidia infect a snail; cercariae develop and are released into the water and penetrate the skin of unwary human swimmers (or waders). Fortunately, humans are not the right host for these parasites and their life cycle ends. Before they die, the cercariae let you know they were present.

After cercariae penetrate the skin, intense pruritus occurs. Five to 10 days later an intensely pruritic rash appears. The patient's rash appears urticarial. The rash can also be papular. If a patient has had a previous exposure, a more intense, papular rash may occur shortly after exposure and persist for 7 to 10 days.

Treatment

Treatment is not necessary to end the infection because humans are not an adequate host for the *Schistosoma* cercariae. If the patient is not tolerating the pruritus, an antihistamine such as diphenhydramine may provide some relief.

Chapter 39

Fever and a Headache

Presentation

An 11-year old arrives in your office with a 1-day history of severe headache and a temperature of 39.1°C (102.4°F). You perform a complete physical examination and find nothing abnormal. He returns to your office 3 days later. The fever and headache have persisted and now he is vomiting and has a generalized maculopapular rash that involves the palms and soles (figures 1–5).

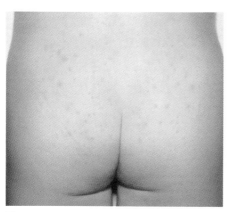

Figure 1

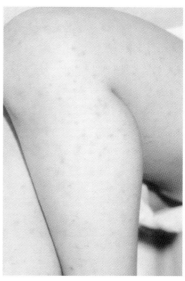

Figure 2

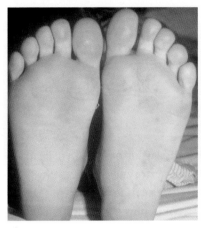

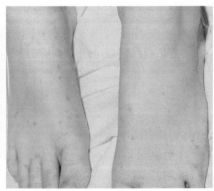

Figure 4

Figure 3

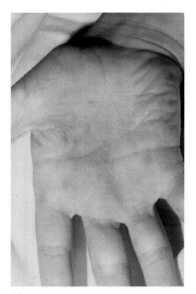

Figure 5

The boy tells you that he lives in the city, but his uncle took him fishing in Fluvanna County in the Rivanna River near their home in Charlottesville, VA. They hiked through the woods to get to his uncle's canoe. When they returned to his uncle's house, the boy checked for ticks when he showered. He did find a few ticks and pulled them straight out with tweezers. However, when he got home, he found an engorged tick in his scalp, which he pulled out. You further discover that his uncle has bird dogs that have the run of his country home. A review of the medical record reveals this boy was one of the first 11-year-olds to get the conjugated tetravalent meningococcal vaccine.

- **What is the diagnosis?**

- **How would you treat this patient?**

Discussion

Diagnosis

You are considering Rocky Mountain spotted fever (RMSF), ehrlichiosis, meningococcemia, and enterovirus infection. Henoch-Schönlein purpura is a possible diagnosis, but the rash is above the umbilicus, involves the palms and soles, and is not purpuric. You consider secondary syphilis, but the patient denies sexual activity. You send blood for culture and send serum to test for RMSF and ehrlichiosis; you begin giving the patient intravenous penicillin and doxycycline.

It is important to recognize and treat RMSF on clinical grounds. You do not want to delay therapy because it will take a while to make a laboratory diagnosis. The history of tick exposure is very important. Unfortunately, lack of tick exposure does not rule out RMSF. The dog tick, *Dermacentor variabilis,* is the tick vector in the south Atlantic, southeast, and south-central states, while *Dermacentor andersoni* is the vector in the northern Rocky Mountain states. The incubation period ranges from 2 to 14 days with an average incubation of 7 days. The erythematous, macular rash usually begins on the ankles and wrists, spreading to involve the limbs and trunk within hours. The rash can become papular and often becomes petechial. The rash is caused by small-vessel vasculitis and usually occurs before the sixth day of illness. The rash is present in about 80% of patients and is a helpful diagnostic feature. Other clinical features include fever, myalgia, severe headache, nausea, vomiting, and anorexia. Patients often have abdominal pain and diarrhea that can mislead the diagnostician. A CBC count might show thrombocytopenia, anemia, or leucopenia. You should also watch for hyponatremia.

Untreated or treated late, RMSF is a dangerous disease that can involve any or all of the major organ systems, resulting in disseminated intravascular coagulation, shock, and death. Lifelong sequelae are not uncommon in RMSF survivors.

A probable diagnosis can be established with a fluorescent antibody titer of 1:64 or higher. A convalescent titer with a fourfold rise over the acute titer is diagnostic.

Treatment
Doxycycline is the drug of choice, even in children younger than 8 years. The risk for dental staining is low with a single course of doxycycline; this is one of those times when effective treatment is more important than the possibility of stained teeth. Furthermore, when the diagnosis is not clear, doxycycline will treat ehrlichia infections; chloramphenicol (another treatment option for RMSF) does not.

Keep in Mind
Get a tick history. Think about the possibility of ehrlichiosis whenever you are considering RMSF in your differential diagnosis. If you think it is RMSF treat with doxycycline. Always think about meningococcemia in a vaccinated patient.

Chapter 40

Fever and Rash Following a Sore Throat

Presentation

An 11-year old girl is brought to your office because of fever, malaise, and headache that began yesterday and the abrupt onset of an erythematous, raised rash on both of her ankles, shins, and knees today. She had a scratchy throat about a week ago, but it lasted only a couple of days; she was well until yesterday. The patient is fully immunized (including hepatitis B virus vaccine) and has never had a serious illness. The family has always lived in suburban Cleveland, has not traveled in the past year, and the 2 siblings and parents are well. There are no pets in the house and neither the mother nor child can recall any ill contacts.

Physical examination reveals a well-developed, cooperative 11-year-old who appears tired. Her temperature is 38.4°C (101°F), respirations are 16 breaths per minute, pulse is 72 beats per minute, and blood pressure is 96/72 mm Hg. There are symmetrical, tender, erythematous, warm nodules and plaques on her ankles, shins, and knees (Figure). The nodules are bright red and raised. There is no popliteal or inguinal lymphadenopathy. There are no other lesions on her skin. Eyes, ears, nose, and throat are normal. Findings from heart, lung, abdominal, musculoskeletal, and neurologic examinations are normal.

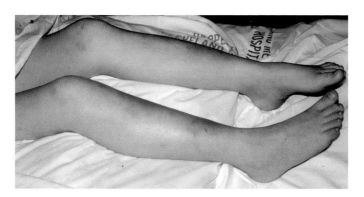

■ **What is your differential diagnosis?**

■ **How will you evaluate this patient?**

■ **How will you manage this patient's disease?**

Discussion

Diagnosis

One of your first thoughts is Henoch-Schönlein purpura, but the lesions are tender and not purpuric and the patient has fever, which is uncommon with Henoch-Schönlein purpura. Your second thought is erythema nodosum. The acute onset of fever and symmetrical, erythematous, tender, raised nodules on the lower extremities fit the clinical diagnosis of erythema nodosum. You recall that erythema nodosum is a hypersensitivity reaction that can be triggered by infections, inflammatory diseases, and drugs. The drugs most commonly implicated as a cause of erythema nodosum are sulfonamides, bromides, and contraceptive pills; your patient has taken none of these.

There is a long list of infections that have been associated with erythema nodosum. Sarcoidosis, although rare in children, is one of the most common diseases associated with erythema nodosum in young adult women. Erythema nodosum also occurs with flares of inflammatory bowel disease, especially ulcerative colitis. Again, this is more common in adults. When tuberculosis was more prevalent it was one of the most common infections associated with erythema nodosum, but this association was seen in only 2 of 62 patients in 2 recent studies of children with erythema nodosum in France and Greece. The most frequent associated infection was group A β-hemolytic streptococci (GABS), which was documented by culture or serology in 23 of the 62 patients reported. Other infections that were documented in the series of children from Greece included *Mycoplasma pneumoniae* (3), *Mycobacterium tuberculosis* (2), *Yersinia enterocolitica* (1), leptospirosis (1), and *Pseudomonas* (1). In the French study, 4 patients had Yersinia infections and 1 each had infections with *Campylobacter* and *Salmonella typhimurium*. Other infections associated with erythema nodosum but not seen in these 2 studies include coccidioidomycosis, histoplasmosis, blastomycosis, syphilis, brucellosis, hepatitis B virus, mononucleosis, leprosy, and *Bartonella henselae.*

Erythema nodosum is usually a clinical diagnosis and a biopsy is not necessary unless the diagnosis is in doubt or the clinical course is atypical. The importance of the workup of a patient with erythema nodosum is to diagnose a treatable underlying disease. The initial laboratory evaluation of a patient with erythema nodosum should include a CBC, erythrocyte sedimentation rate (ESR), antistreptolysin O (ASO) titer, throat culture, intradermal tuberculin skin test (TST), stool culture (if there is a history of diarrhea), and a chest x-ray film. The CBC is usually normal or shows a slightly elevated WBC count. The ESR can be very high, and in children there is often a direct correlation between the number of lesions and the level of the ESR. An elevated ASO titer is suggestive of a recent GABS infection, and a positive result from throat culture is diagnostic. Stool culture from a patient with recent or current diarrhea may identify one of the related enteric pathogens mentioned previously. A through history for exposure to tuberculosis should be obtained, but even if the history is negative, a TST should be placed and read at 48 to 72 hours. The chest x-ray film is obtained to rule out sarcoidosis (which was diagnosed in 4 of the 32 cases reported in France). The decision to evaluate for other infectious diseases should be based on clues in the history or clinical signs and symptoms. In this case, you decide to test for Epstein-Barr virus mononucleosis, but because the girl has been immunized against hepatitis B and has no risk factors, you do not test for hepatitis B. There is no reason to suspect a fungal infection or leprosy.

Your patient has a normal CBC and differential count. Her ESR is 88 mm/h. Throat culture is negative for GABS and her ASO titer in not elevated. Epstein-Barr virus serology is negative and her chest x-ray is normal. There is no reaction to the TST at 48 or 72 hours. You give the patient acetaminophen for pain. Over 3 days of observation the lesions flatten out and take on a purplish color. The patient defervesces and is feeling better. The lesions are no longer warm or painful. You elect to continue to observe the patient without further evaluation. One week after presentation the lesions are a yellowish color and appear similar to a resolving, deep bruise. Two weeks after presentation the lesions have resolved and the patient is well. You tell the family that even though the trigger for this episode of erythema nodosum was not discovered, it is unlikely that she will have another episode.

Keep in Mind

Erythema nodosum is a self-limited hypersensitivity reaction, but many of the diseases that can trigger erythema nodosum are not. Many of the infectious triggers can be treated and systemic diseases such as sarcoidosis and inflammatory bowel disease will require long-term management. Erythema nodosum has also been seen in patients subsequently diagnosed with lymphoma.

Chapter 41

Pearly Papules

Presentation

An 11-year-old boy in your office is upset about a rash on his face that started more than 2 months ago and is not clearing up (Figure). He thinks it is getting worse. The rash is entirely benign and the patient's concerns center on his appearance. The patient is in excellent health and has never been seriously ill. He has never had skin problems before and no one in his family has lesions similar to his.

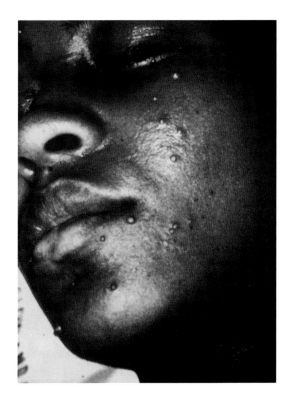

The findings from the physical examination are normal except for approximately 20 pearly pink-to-white, dome-shaped papules with a smooth surface. Some of the lesions have central umbilication. There are minimal to no signs of inflammation surrounding the lesions. The lesions range from 1 to 5 mm in diameter and are firm to palpation. Although he does have papules on his eyelids, his conjunctivae are clear.

- ■ **What is your diagnosis?**

- ■ **Do you want to perform any diagnostic tests?**

- ■ **How will you treat this patient?**

Discussion

Diagnosis

The presence of asymptomatic, pearly papules with umbilicated centers for several weeks is diagnostic for molluscum contagiosum. Molluscum contagiosum is caused by *Molluscipoxvirus,* a member of the poxvirus family. The infection is spread by contact with infected people or contaminated objects or by autoinoculation. Only humans can be infected by *Molluscipoxvirus.* Molluscum contagiosum is seen worldwide and occurs most commonly in school-aged children. The virus has an incubation period of 2 weeks to 6 months. The infection is uncommon in children younger than 1 year. This can probably be explained by the presence of maternal antibodies and the long incubation period. The lesions of molluscum contagiosum are most commonly found on the face, trunk, and extremities. Genital involvement without sexual contact is not uncommon. Nonetheless, the presence of genital molluscum contagiosum in a child should raise the possibility of sexual abuse. Conjunctivitis may be present in patients with lesions on their eyelids. Rarely, the virus can directly infect the bulbar conjunctivae or cornea. If you suspect eye involvement, the patient should be seen by a pediatric ophthalmologist.

Treatment

Molluscum contagiosum is a self-limited disease. Untreated, lesions will eventually resolve on their own in immunocompetent patients. An individual lesion resolves in about 2 months and all lesions will usually resolve in 6 to 9 months. Because lesions are usually asymptomatic, almost any treatment will cause more discomfort to the patient than the lesions themselves. Physical injury to individual lesions with cryosurgery and curettage is the most common treatment. Many chemical treatments have been tried with varying success, including podophyllin, cantharidin, trichloroacetic acid, phenol, and salicylic acid. A dermatologist should be consulted before undertaking the treatment of large lesions or patients with numerous lesions or lesions in difficult places to treat. You advise this boy and his family to wait a few more weeks before undertaking a therapy that might result in more scarring than would be caused by allowing the lesions to resolve on their own. The family agrees to see you again in 4 weeks before making a treatment decision.

Keep in Mind

Primum non nocere—first do no harm.

Part 4

Case Reports in Teenagers

Chapter 42

Red Plaque

Presentation

A 14-year-old boy is in your office because he has a ring-shaped lesion on his left forearm. The lesion started as a red plaque that gradually has increased in size. At his mother's suggestion, he applied an over-the-counter preparation of 0.5% hydrocortisone cream. The redness and itching decreased when he applied the hydrocortisone cream, only to reappear when he stopped applying it. He is otherwise healthy and has no other complaints. No one in his family and none of his friends have similar lesions. His past medical, family, and social histories are non-contributory. Findings from a review of systems are negative.

On physical examination you see a lesion about the size of a half-dollar, red and raised at the border with central clearing and scaling (Figure 1). There are no other lesions on his body.

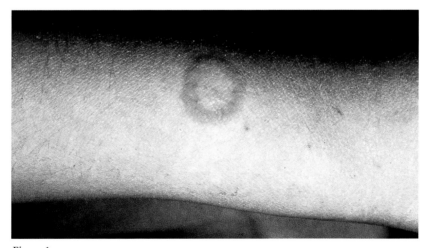

Figure 1

■ **What is your differential diagnosis?**

■ **What laboratory tests would you obtain?**

■ **How will you treat this patient?**

Discussion

Diagnosis

The lesion looks like tinea corporis (ringworm), but you consider other diseases that can produce similar lesions. Nummular eczema can produce scaly annular plaques that persist for weeks to months. Patients with nummular eczema usually have multiple lesions and a history of atopy or xeroderma. Urticaria can also take this shape, but the lesions are edematous and last for hours or days, not weeks. Erythema migrans (Lyme disease) enlarges rapidly with central clearing. Erythema migrans lesions are usually solitary and are accompanied by fever, arthralgia, myalgia, malaise, and a history of a tick bite (see Chapter 36). Granuloma annulare lesions are pink to violaceous, solitary or multiple, and usually on the distal extremities or hands and feet. The herald lesion of pityriasis rosea also can be annular with central clearing, but the patient will develop a more generalized rash on the trunk within a few days of the herald patch. Having done this useful mental exercise, you conclude that tinea corporis is the most likely diagnosis and elect to treat empirically.

If you were less certain you could gently scrape scale from the active border of the lesion onto a glass slide, add a drop of potassium hydroxide, gently heat, and look for fungal hyphae under a light microscope. A negative potassium hydroxide preparation does not rule out a dermatophyte infection. Scale can also be inoculated directly onto dermatophyte test medium culture and incubated at room temperature. After 1 to 2 weeks, a phenol red indicator in the agar will turn from yellow to red in the area surrounding a dermatophyte colony. A third option would be to send a specimen of scrapings to a microbiology laboratory for culture on Sabouraud dextrose agar.

Treatment

For limited infections such as the one your patient has, there are a wide variety of options for topical therapy, including miconazole nitrate, clotrimazole, terbinafine, tolnaftate, naftifine hydrochloride, or ciclopirox olamine twice a day, or ketoconazole, econazole nitrate, oxiconazole nitrate, butenafine hydrochloride, or sulconazole nitrate once a day. Topical treatment should be continued for 1 to 2 weeks after the lesion has cleared visually. For more widespread infections, systemic griseofulvin remains the drug of choice.

Keep in Mind

Other causes of ring-shaped lesions that you should consider before treating for tinea corporis are pityriasis rosea and nummular eczema (figures 2 and 3).

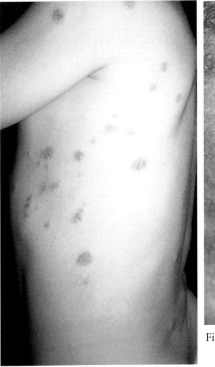

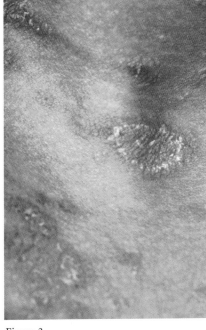

Figure 3

Figure 2

Chapter 43

Fever, Arthritis, and Dermatitis

Presentation

A 16-year-old girl is in your office today because of scattered lesions on her arms, legs, hands, and feet. She also reports pain and swelling in both knees and left wrist. She explains that she first noticed mild pain and swelling in her left knee about 4 days ago. The next day she had pain and swelling in her left wrist and today noted the skin lesions. You ask her if she has had a fever and she replies that she has not taken her temperature, but has felt warmer than usual. The patient is fully immunized and has never been seriously ill. Menarche began when she was 10 years old and she currently has regular periods with a 28-day cycle. Her last menstrual period ended 2 days ago. She denies being sexually active. Her past medical and family histories are noncontributory. She was an A and B student through junior high school, but her grades fell to Bs and Cs as a freshman and she is currently failing 2 of her 5 subjects as a sophomore. Her mother says she is friends with a group of teens who reportedly have been drinking alcohol and smoking marijuana. The parents have encouraged their daughter to see a counselor, but she refuses.

The patient is a well developed, mature-looking 16-year-old who does not appear to be acutely ill. Her vital signs are normal except for her temperature, which is 38°C (100.4°F). Examination of her skin reveals discrete papules and pustules on her extremities including her hands and feet, fore-arms, and shins (figures 1 and 2). The papular lesions are erythematous, but not painful to touch. There are about a dozen lesions total.

You find a solitary hemorrhagic lesion on her left foot (Figure 3)

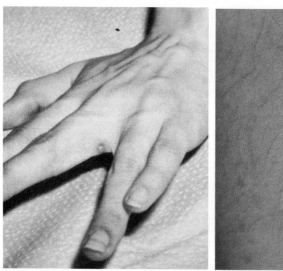

Figure 1

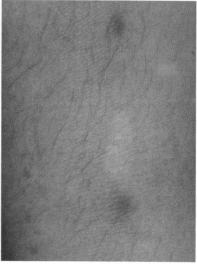

Figure 2

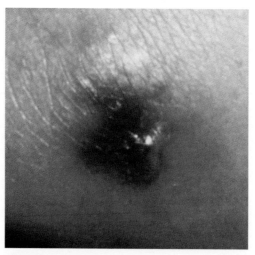

Figure 3

Her eyes, ears, nose, and throat are normal. Examination of the nail-fold capillaries using your ophthalmoscope shows a normal capillary pattern (see figures 2 and 3 in Chapter 21). She has no cervical, axillary, or inguinal lymphadenopathy. Her lungs are clear and she does not have a murmur. Her external genital examination reveals that she is Tanner stage 5 and there is no vaginal discharge. Examination of both knees and the left wrist reveal mild swelling and pain on movement of the joints. The results of her neurologic examination are normal and she does not have signs of meningeal irritation.

- ■ **What is your differential diagnosis?**

- ■ **What information is missing from this history?**

- ■ **What diagnostic tests would you like to perform?**

- ■ **How will you manage the disease?**

Discussion

Diagnosis
Your most pressing concern is the possibility that this patient could have meningococcemia. However, a 4-day illness with a pustular, papular rash, rather than petechial, in a patient who does not appear very ill makes you think that meningococcemia is unlikely. Chronic meningococcemia is a possibility, but does not require immediate intervention. You also consider the possibility of inflammatory arthritis. Normal capillary nail-fold examination does not rule out this possibility. Reiter syndrome is characterized by urethritis, cervicitis, and skin lesions that are sometimes pustular. The absence of mucosal lesions makes Reiter syndrome less likely. Infectious carditis is possible, but the patient does not have a predisposing condition, use intravenous drugs, or have a murmur. Infectious arthritis is also possible, but usually does not involve multiple joints. The combination of a low-grade fever, additive joint involvement with an asymmetric distribution, and a papulopustular rash on the extremities makes you think that this teen may have disseminated gonococcal infection (DGI). She denied being sexually active, but her mother was in the room.

You ask the mother for permission to speak to the patient alone. You explain to the patient that you are almost certain that she has a sexually transmitted infection and you need to know her true sexual history. You also tell her that it will be important for her partners to be checked and treated. She now admits that when she is drinking and smoking marijuana with her friends, she has been having sex as well. There are 3 or 4 boys in the group that she has had sex with over the past year. Condoms are seldom used. The last time she had intercourse was about a week ago. None of her friends have said anything about having a sexually transmitted infection. You ask the mother to return to the room and explain that you suspect that her daughter has DGI and tell her that the patient will need to be hospitalized for further evaluation and treatment. You recommend that the patient be admitted to the care of the adolescent medicine specialist; the patient and her mother agree. You call the adolescent medicine doctor and she agrees to accept the patient. She asks you to send the patient to the emergency department (ED) where it will be easier to perform a complete pelvic examination.

The adolescent medicine physician meets the patient in the ED where she confirms your findings and performs a bimanual and speculum pelvic examination. There is no adnexal or cervical tenderness, the cervix does not appear inflamed, and there is no cervical discharge. Nonetheless, a cervical swab specimen is obtained for Gram stain and culture. A specimen of blood is obtained for a CBC and culture. The left knee is aspirated and approximately 10 mL of straw-colored fluid is obtained and sent for a cell count and culture. The patient is given 1 g of ceftriaxone by the intramuscular route and oral doxycycline to treat a possible *Chlamydia* infection, then admitted to the adolescent unit. The CBC result is normal and the synovial fluid has 12,000 WBCs/μL. Cultures of blood and synovial fluid are sterile. *Neisseria gonorrhoeae* is cultured from the cervical swab specimen and is determined to be susceptible to penicillin. The local health department is notified. On the second hospital day the patient is afebrile and has no new skin lesions; the original skin lesions are beginning to resolve. Her knees and wrist are less painful and the swelling has diminished.

People with DGI often have fever, granulocytosis, and signs of systemic toxicity like malaise and headache. Signs and symptoms tend to be mild. Blood culture results from patients with DGI will be positive about 50% of the time and cultures of synovial fluid are usually sterile unless the patient has infective arthritis. Results from culture and Gram stain of skin lesions are positive 10% to 15% of the time. When DGI is suspected at least 3 blood cultures should be obtained and synovial fluid should be cultured when it can be obtained. Cultures should also be obtained from the urethra or endocervix, rectum, and pharynx because *N gonorrhoeae* can be isolated from a mucosal site in about 80% of patients. Infective endocarditis occurs in about 1% to 2% of patients with DGI.

Treatment
Patients with DGI should be treated with intravenous or intramuscular ceftriaxone or with another intravenous third-generation cephalosporin. If the patient does not have septic arthritis or other complications, the patient may be changed to an oral regimen when there are clear signs of clinical improvement. Oral therapy can be tailored based on susceptibility testing. In this patient oral penicillin therapy would be an option. If no organism has been isolated, oral cefixime or ciprofloxacin should be given to complete a total of 7 to 10 days of antibacterial therapy. All patients with gonococcal infections should be treated for *Chlamydia* as well.

Keep in Mind
If the history does not fit the clinical signs and symptoms, there is a good chance that the history might be inaccurate. Obtaining an accurate sexual history from a teen can be a challenge; adolescent medicine specialists can offer valuable help and guidance. Don't forget to test for *Chlamydia*, syphilis, and human immunodeficiency virus infections.

Chapter 44

Fatigue, Lethargy, and Erythema

Presentation

A 16-year-old girl comes to your office on Monday morning because she has been tired and has not had her usual appetite for the past 2 weeks. Initially, she had a cough, headache, and nausea, but she did not have a fever. Although no one else in the family was ill, influenza is circulating in the community and several of her high school classmates have had the flu. You have seen many patients with influenza in your practice.

On physical examination she appears weak and gives curt answers to your questions. She is afebrile with a normal pulse and respiratory rate, but her blood pressure is 140/90 mm Hg. You also detect erythema and swelling of her hands and feet and her lips are erythematous. The findings of the remainder of the physical examination are normal.

You believe her illness is most likely influenza with some atypical features, or possibly Epstein-Barr virus mononucleosis. The swelling of her hands and feet and her red lips bring to mind Kawasaki disease, but the lack of fever and her age cause you to dismiss this diagnosis.

You are concerned about her elevated blood pressure. You obtain a CBC, electrolytes, blood urea nitrogen (BUN), creatinine, and an urinalysis, of which the findings from all are normal. A monospot test is negative. The results of the laboratory tests are reassuring and you advise the family that the patient probably has a bad case of influenza and should start feeling better over the next few days. You instruct them to return if she is not better within 1 week.

She returns to your office on Friday. She says she is even more tired, still has no appetite, and her hands and feet have become pruritic and are desquamating. She complains of severe pain in her wrists and legs that is not relieved by acetaminophen. On examination her blood pressure remains elevated at 140/90 mm Hg and she has lost 2 kg since Monday. She appears ill. Her lips remain erythematous and her hands and feet are notable for erythema and desquamation (Figure). Eyes, ears, nose, and throat are normal, as are the heart and lungs. Her abdomen is soft, there are no masses, and the liver and spleen are not enlarged. She does not have any enlarged lymph nodes, and findings of joint and neurologic examinations are normal. The only thing you are sure about is that this teen is ill and needs to be hospitalized for further evaluation.

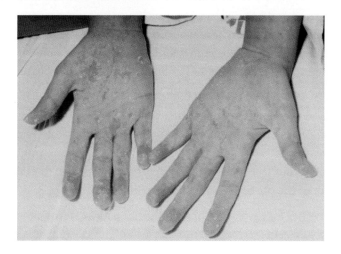

- ■ **What is your differential diagnosis?**

- ■ **Is there more information that you would like from the history?**

- ■ **How will you evaluate this patient's condition further?**

Discussion

Diagnosis

You are faced with a 16-year-old girl with a 3-week history of fatigue, irritability, weight loss, swelling, redness and desquamation of the hands and feet, erythema of the lips, pain in the wrists and legs, and hypertension. The most striking physical finding is the desquamation on the hands and feet. Diseases that result in desquamation during the convalescent stage include Kawasaki disease, scarlet fever, staphylococcal scalded skin syndrome, and streptococcal and staphylococcal toxic shock syndromes. Her age coupled with no fever, no conjunctivitis, and no rash make typical Kawasaki disease unlikely. Her clinical course argues against a bacterial infection and makes most infectious diseases unlikely. The other major clue from physical examination is her elevated blood pressure. You consider the possibility that she could have a malignancy like pheochromocytoma, a connective tissue disease like dermatomyositis, a drug reaction, or some kind of intoxication.

You review the history and ask about all medications she has taken, but she denies having taken anything except acetaminophen. She has not experimented with any drugs and has not tried any home remedies. You repeat the CBC, electrolytes, creatinine, BUN, and urinalysis and obtain an erythrocyte sedimentation rate (ESR). All are normal; the ESR is 4 mm/h. You consult cardiology to rule out atypical Kawasaki disease; the echocardiogram is normal. You consult nephrology to evaluate and treat her hypertension. Her serum renin concentration is slightly increased at 3 ng/(L · sec) (normal is 0–2.8 ng/[L · sec]) and her serum norepinephrine and epinephrine levels are elevated. Abdominal ultrasound and CT scans with contrast of the abdomen, chest, head, and neck fail to identify a tumor or any structural abnormality of the kidneys. Blood pressure control requires multiple antihypertensive agents. The rheumatologist does not think this is a connective tissues disease based on the history and physical findings and normal ESR, but suggests that you check her creatinine phosphokinase levels; they are within normal limits. Dermatology is consulted. On the basis of erythema of the lips, pruritus, erythema, swelling of the hands and feet, and the negative workup, the dermatologist suggests the possibility of mercury poisoning.

You ask the patient about possible exposure to mercury. About a week before she came down with the "flu" a barometer that she had used for a science project fell from her bedroom wall and broke. She cleaned up the mess as best she could, but did not report the accident to her parents. Her urine mercury concentration is markedly elevated.

The type of mercury exposure determines the clinical syndromes associated with mercury intoxication. Elemental mercury is only negligibly absorbed by the skin or gastrointestinal tract; intoxication occurs by inhaling mercury vapor when mercury is oxidized to mercuric ion by exposure to oxygen. Acute exposure to large doses of mercury vapor produces acute damage to the lungs, skin, eyes, and gingiva and patients present with cough, chest pain, rash, conjunctivitis, fever, nausea, and vomiting. Hypertension has been consistently reported and can mimic pheochromocytoma. It has been suggested that this is related to mercury-binding S-adenosylmethionine, which is required to convert norepinephrine to epinephrine. Thus, norepinephrine, epinephrine, and dopamine accumulate, mimicking the signs and symptoms of a pheochromocytoma.

Chronic exposure to lower doses of mercury can result in central and peripheral nervous system signs such as tremors, irritability, and emotional lability in addition to anorexia, headaches, weakness, malaise, and muscle pain. Sources of elemental mercury include instruments such as thermometers and barometers, alkaline batteries, neon lights, paint, dental amalgams, and herbal preparations containing mercury.

Methylmercury poisoning from the ingestion of contaminated fish has garnered much attention in the press in recent years. Methylmercury poisoning has a delayed onset and manifests as neurotoxicity. The wide array of signs and symptoms associated with methylmercury intoxication include ataxia; dysarthria; paresthesias; tremors; movement disorders; impairment of vision, hearing, taste, and smell; memory loss; dementia; and death. In utero exposure can result in microcephaly, developmental delay, deafness, blindness, and seizures.

Pink disease, also known as acrodynia, is a hypersensitivity reaction to elemental mercury that is seen primarily in children. Methylmercury intoxication does not result in acrodynia. Pink disease is characterized by severe pain and a papular, pruritic, pink rash on the extremities, including the hands and feet and possibly the face. Children with pink disease may also be anorectic and apathetic and have hypotonia of the pectoral and pelvic muscle groups.

Treatment
The treatment of mercury poisoning requires removing the source of exposure, providing supportive therapy, and removing the mercury from the body. Patients should not receive chelation therapy unless blood or urine concentrations of mercury are extremely elevated. Chelation is most effective for the removal of elemental mercury and least effective for the removal of methylmercury. The agents that are recommended are 2,3-dimercaptosuccinic acid (DMSA) or 2,3-dimercapto-1-propane sulfonic acid (DMPS); either can be administered orally. Chelation should not be undertaken without consultation with a medical toxicologist.

The prognosis for mercury intoxication is guarded, as neurologic sequelae may be permanent.

Keep in Mind
Clues in evaluating hard-to-diagnose patients may not be obvious to the patient or family. Sometimes the clinical findings require us to ask about unusual exposures.

Chapter 45

Fever, Malaise, and Nodules

Presentation

A previously healthy 13-year-old boy is in your office because he has had fever, malaise, and easy fatigability for the past 5 days. You have been this boy's pediatrician since birth; he is fully immunized and has never had a serious illness. It has been more than 2 years since his last sick visit.

On physical examination the patient appears ill. His temperature is 39°C (102.2°F), pulse is 96 beats per minute, respiratory rate is 16 breaths per minute, and blood pressure is 100/70 mm Hg. Examination of the skin reveals several pea-sized, moveable, non-tender masses over the extensor surface of his elbows (Figure 1) and on the dorsum of the middle finger of his right hand (Figure 2). The masses are not pruritic and there is no rash. Eyes, ears, nose, and throat are normal and he does not have lymphadenopathy. Auscultation of the heart reveals a grade 3/6 high-frequency, blowing, apical holosystolic murmur and a lower pitched, mid-diastolic apical murmur. Peripheral pulses are normal. His lungs are clear, his liver and spleen are normal, and no abdominal mass is palpated. The findings from the musculoskeletal and neurologic examinations are normal.

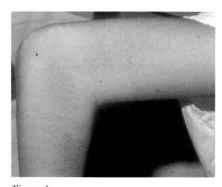

Figure 1

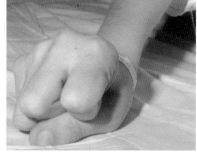

Figure 2

- **What questions would you like to ask this patient or his parents?**

- **What are your major diagnostic considerations?**

- **What diagnostic tests would you obtain?**

- **How will you treat this teen?**

Discussion

Diagnosis

The most worrisome finding on physical examination is the heart murmur. You quickly check his medical record to confirm your recollection that you have never heard a murmur in this patient before. You ask the parents whether anyone else has told them that their son has a heart murmur and they reply in the negative. The patient also denies having a sore throat in the past 3 to 4 weeks, joint swelling or pain, or a rash. Although the murmur could be caused by viral myopericarditis or bacterial endocarditis, you are most concerned about rheumatic fever. The murmur does not sound like a functional murmur and it is unlikely for a murmur associated with congenital heart disease to be showing up now. The skin masses also fit with descriptions of the subcutaneous nodules that are one of the major Jones criteria in the diagnosis of rheumatic fever. You obtain a throat culture for group A β-hemolytic streptococci (GABS), draw a specimen of blood to send for an erythrocyte sedimentation rate (ESR) and antibody titers to streptococcal extracellular products (streptolysin O, streptokinase, hyaluronidase, deoxyribonuclease, and nicotinamide adenine di-nucleotidase), and call the pediatric cardiologist. After you review the case on the phone, the cardiologist tells you to send the patient to her office today for examination and an echocardiogram.

After the cardiologist examines the boy, she calls to tell you that your patient has mitral insufficiency. The mitral valve leaflets are thickened and there is incomplete closure of the valve. She also tells you that the left atrium and ventricle are dilated. These findings coupled with the cutaneous nodules make the diagnosis of acute rheumatic fever likely.

Rheumatic fever follows an antecedent GABS infection by 3 to 4 weeks. The pathogenesis remains unclear, but it is thought that the immune response to certain strains of GABS in genetically susceptible hosts is responsible for the clinical manifestations. Rheumatic fever is a self-limited disease that can affect the heart, brain, joints, and skin. Damage to the heart is the only potential long-term sequelae.

The diagnosis of rheumatic fever generally requires that the patient meet 2 of the major Jones criteria or 1 major criterion and 2 minor criteria plus evidence of a previous GABS infection. Boxes 1 and 2 list major and minor Jones criteria.

Box 1. Major Jones Criteria	Box 2. Minor Jones Criteria
Polyarthritis Carditis Chorea Erythema marginatum Subcutaneous nodules	Fever Arthralgia Elevated ESR or CRP Prolonged PR interval Previous rheumatic fever or rheumatic heart disease

Supporting evidence of a previous GABS infection includes a positive throat culture for GABS, increased antistreptolysin O (ASO) or other streptococcal antibodies, or recent scarlet fever.

Polyarthritis occurs in about 70% of patients with rheumatic fever. The arthritis begins abruptly with pain, swelling, warmth, and redness of the involved joints. It usually involves large joints, most commonly affecting the knees, elbows, ankles, and wrists. The arthritis migrates from joint to joint and responds to treatment with salicylate within 24 to 48 hours. Rheumatic fever does not cause permanent joint damage and persistence of arthritis or arthralgia beyond the acute phase of the disease should make you doubt the diagnosis.

Carditis occurs in about 50% of rheumatic fever patients and is responsible for most of the morbidity and mortality associated with the disease.

Although carditis can involve the endocardium, myocardium, or peri-
cardium, endocardial involvement with evidence of mitral or aortic valve
insufficiency is required to diagnose rheumatic fever.

Sydenham chorea has been reported in 5% to 30% of patients with rheumatic fever. Chorea may be a late or the only manifestation of rheumatic
fever. Chorea usually occurs 2 months or more after the GABS infection
and there may be no other evidence of rheumatic fever. Involuntary, pur-
poseless movements of facial and skeletal muscles characterize Sydenham
chorea. Patients may also experience weakness and emotional lability.
Deterioration in handwriting, a so-called milkmaid grip, and spooning of
the fingers are also used to characterize Sydenham chorea. Chorea usually
subsides within 2 months, but may recur.

Erythema marginatum and subcutaneous nodules are rare manifestations
of rheumatic fever, occurring in fewer than 5% of cases. Erythema marginatum (Figure 3) begins as pink macules or papules that expand into
annular plaques with pale centers. The border is usually distinct and
expands rapidly to form rings. Although the lesions can appear urticarial,
they are not pruritic. The rash is typically on the trunk and proximal
extremities; it is evanescent and may go unnoticed by the patient. The
rash is seen most commonly at the time when arthritis or carditis is most
severe and only lasts for 1 or 2 days. The lesions may appear after a warm
bath or shower.

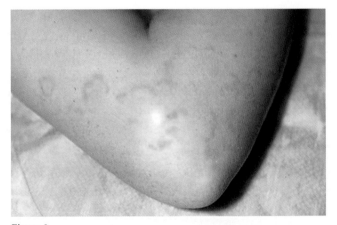

Figure 3

Subcutaneous nodules are pea-sized masses that appear over the extensor surfaces of the elbows, wrists, and knees and less commonly over the spine and suboccipital areas. The masses are firm, non-tender, and moveable. Subcutaneous nodules usually are observed in patients with the most severe forms of carditis.

Patients with rheumatic fever usually have a temperature of 39°C (102.2°F) at the time of presentation. Patients who present with Sydenham chorea are usually afebrile. Arthralgia is pain limited to joints without evidence of inflammation. The ESR and CRP are usually elevated in patients with acute rheumatic fever. Patients presenting with chorea usually have normal acute phase reactants. A prolonged PR interval on the electrocardiogram is common and serves as a minor criterion, but is not diagnostic of carditis.

Treatment

The treatment of acute rheumatic fever is directed at eliminating any residual GABS infection and treating the acute inflammatory process. Penicillin continues to be the drug of choice for treating GABS and aspirin the drug of choice for treating inflammation. Patients with carditis should continue aspirin therapy for 6 to 8 weeks. Approximately 3 to 4 weeks of aspirin therapy is usually adequate for patients without carditis. It is helpful to track the ESR in patients with and without carditis; continue aspirin therapy until the ESR has begun to normalize. If signs or symptoms recur, aspirin therapy should be reinstituted.

To prevent recurrent attacks of rheumatic fever, long-term penicillin prophylaxis should be instituted. Patients with carditis and residual heart disease should continue prophylaxis for 10 years after the last episode or until the patient is 40 years of age, whichever is longer. For patients with carditis but no residual heart disease, penicillin should be continued for 10 years or well into adulthood, whichever is longer. Patients without carditis should be given penicillin for 5 years or until the age of 21 years, whichever is longer.

Keep in Mind

Reye syndrome occurs in patients with influenza or varicella who receive aspirin. To avoid Reye syndrome, patients with rheumatic fever on long-term aspirin therapy should be vaccinated against chickenpox unless a history of chickenpox disease is confirmed.

Patients with rheumatic fever should receive influenza vaccine or, if diagnosed with rheumatic fever during the influenza season, prophylactic antiviral therapy.

Rheumatic fever continues to be a complication of GABS pharyngitis and should be part of the differential diagnosis of any patient with fever, arthritis, or new murmur, as well as patients with onset of choreoathetoid movements.

Chapter 46

Persistent Arm Nodule

Presentation

A 16-year-old girl visits your office for what she describes as a boil on the upper-outer area of her left arm. The patient noticed a pruritic papule in the same place about 2 weeks ago. At that time she was nearing the end of a 2-week trip to Belize with a church group to help in the construction of a school. The pruritus stopped after 1 or 2 days and the papule on her arm did not bother her over the next week. About 1 week ago the papule began to enlarge and developed a central pore that sometimes discharged a brownish fluid. Most of the time the lesion was not really painful, but every few days she would experience a sharp pain. She says that it almost feels like something is moving inside of the lesion.

You have been this girl's pediatrician since her birth and know her past medical history and review of systems to be noncontributory.

The findings from the physical examination are normal except for the lesion on her left arm. The lesion is a 1.2-cm, firm, red, non-tender nodule in the subcutaneous tissue above the triceps muscle. It does not feel fluctuant and when you gently apply pressure to the nodule, there is no discharge from what appears to be a central opening (Figure 1).

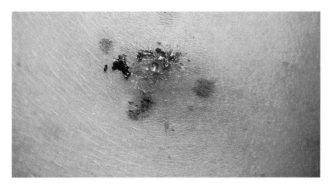

Figure 1

You tell the girl and her parents that you think this is an infected insect bite. The size of the lesion and its progression over 2 weeks lead you to prescribe a 1-week course of cephalexin.

One week later the girl is back in your office and the lesion is unchanged. However, the patient has made a disconcerting observation. She decided to put triple antibacterial ointment on the lesion in addition to taking the cephalexin you prescribed. She tells you that within 1 hour of putting the ointment on the lesion she feels something moving and can see something white sticking out of the center of the lesion. When she tries to pick at the lesion, the white thing in the center disappears.

- **What is the diagnosis?**
- **What diagnostic tests will you order?**
- **How will you treat this patient's condition?**

Discussion

Diagnosis

You take what your patient tells you seriously and ask the patient and her mother if they are willing to put antibacterial ointment on the lesion and wait in the waiting room until the change she has described occurs. They agree. You instruct your staff to put the patient in an examination room as soon as she sees anything protruding from the center of the lesion. About an hour later you are told that the patient is in an examination room and there is indeed something white in the center of the lesion. On inspection you observe a bobbing form in the opening of the nodule. This appears to be some type of parasite and you are not sure how you should proceed. You call the pediatric infectious disease specialist and tell him the story. The ID specialist thinks the patient may have myiasis and what you are looking at may be the larva of a botfly. He suggests 2 possibilities—grasp the white material protruding from the center of the lesion with tweezers and remove it, or put more ointment on the lesion, cover it with gauze, and send the patient to the emergency department (ED), where he will see the patient.

You feel more comfortable with the second suggestion and send the patient to the ED.

When the ID specialist sees the patient in the ED, the lesion has been covered with ointment for nearly 3 hours and with the gauze for nearly 2 hours. The ID specialist confirms the history and gently removes the gauze with tweezers in hand to grasp the protruding larva. The larva is partially enmeshed in the gauze and is unable to make a hasty retreat back into the nodular lesion. The doctor grasps the larva with tweezers and gently pulls out an intact *Dermatobia hominis* larva that is more than 1 cm long (Figure 2). The doctor tells the patient and her mother that removal of the larva is curative and the lesion should heal completely without any further intervention.

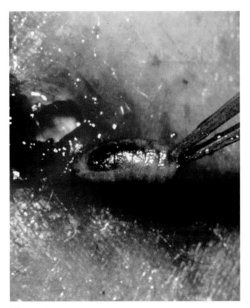

Figure 2

The ID specialist calls you back to let you know that he has removed the larva and the patient should be fine. He also tells you what he knows about furuncular myiasis caused by botfly infestation. The human botfly, *Dermatobia hominis,* inhabits forests from Central Mexico to Argentina.

The female fly attaches her eggs to the underside of mosquitoes, biting flies, or ticks while in mid-flight. When these vectors feed on humans or other animals, fly larvae emerge from the eggs and invade the skin. Each larva produces a separate lesion. A nodular lesion develops in which the larva grows over a period of 6 to 12 weeks, reaching a size of 18 to 24 mm. The nodule will have a central aperture through which the larva will often protrude. Occlusion of the aperture is one of the less invasive ways to remove the larva. Applying bacon fat to cover the central aperture is a safe and simple way to facilitate removal of larvae.

The differential diagnosis of furuncular myiasis includes cellulitis, sebaceous cysts, and staphylococcal boils. Myiasis should be considered in patients who have a non-healing nodular skin lesion and have been to an area where the human botfly is endemic.

Treatment is removal of the larva. It is best to remove the larva intact because retained parts of the larva can cause ongoing inflammation. Compressing the nodule to expel the larva is not advised. If necessary, the larva can be removed surgically.

Keep in Mind
As more people travel, we are likely to see infections that were not part of our medical training. Careful history taking and observation usually will provide the answer.

Chapter 47

Stabbing Abdominal Pain

Presentation

A 14-year-old girl visits your office because of severe abdominal pain that is "stabbing" in nature. It is not relieved by extra-strength acetaminophen, but is somewhat relieved when the girl sleeps on her left side. She was entirely well until 3 days ago when she began to have periumbilical pain that moved to her right lower quadrant. She has not been eating or drinking well and her urine output has been lower than usual. She has not had a bowel movement in 4 days. Her oral temperature last night was between 39.4°C (102.9°F) and 40°C (104°F) and she has had a headache for the past 2 days. She denies nausea or vomiting. Her history for possible exposure to infectious agents is negative, except she does tell you that she drank unpasteurized milk while visiting relatives at their farm last week.

On physical examination you find a developmentally appropriate 14-year-old who is in mild distress. Her vital signs, including her temperature, are normal. She has mild periumbilical tenderness to palpation. She also is tender in the right lower quadrant over the McBurney point. There is no rebound tenderness, nor is there tenderness on digital rectal examination. Stool on the examining glove was positive for occult blood. You think this could be appendicitis and you telephone the pediatric surgeon on call, who asks you to send the patient to the local emergency department for examination and admission.

The surgeon agrees that this could be a surgical abdomen and orders a CT scan of the abdomen. The scan shows nonspecific, abnormal thickening of the wall of the cecum and the entire right side of the colon (Figure 1). Free fluid is present in the pelvis. The terminal ileum appears to have subtle wall thickening. The appendix and uterus are normal. The radiologist tells you that it looks like inflammatory bowel disease (IBD), but he cannot rule out an infectious etiology.

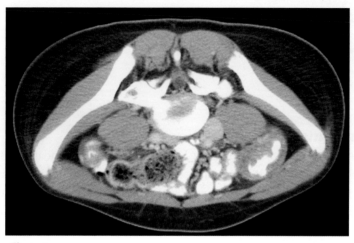

Figure 1

- **What is your differential diagnosis based on this information?**

- **What tests would you order to narrow the possibilities?**

- **Is there anything you want to treat before you get test results?**

Discussion

Diagnosis

While you were taking the patient's history you considered the possibility of an ectopic pregnancy, an ovarian cyst, or torsion of an ovary, but after you examined the patient you were more concerned about the gastrointestinal tract than the genitourinary system. In fact, when you called your surgical colleague you were fairly certain the diagnosis was appendicitis. He agreed—until the results of the abdominal CT scan came back showing a normal appendix. Because the patient has not had a bowel movement in 4 days, gastroenteritis does not seem very likely. The radiologist thinks the bowel thickening looks more like IBD than an infection (but he is not willing to rule out infection).

The CBC shows 22,500 WBCs/µL with 15% bands. The metabolic screen results are within normal limits. The patient's temperature rose to 39.6°C (103.3°F) after admission, so you obtained blood to send for culture. You want to culture her stool, but there is none to culture. Thinking that this may be IBD, you consult the pediatric gastroenterologist. When he hears about the unpasteurized milk ingestion, he suggests waiting until stool culture results are available before further evaluating for IBD. You give the patient a laxative and wait.

Your patient begins having 6 to 8 watery stools a day, more than enough to culture. She does not see blood or mucus mixed with her stool, but does notice blood on the toilet paper sometimes. The blood culture is positive for gram-negative rods before stool culture results are available and you begin therapy with intravenous gentamicin. You visit the microbiology

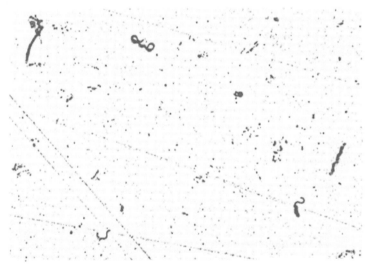

Figure 2 (Courtesy of William A. Clark, MD, Centers for Disease Control and Prevention, Atlanta, GA)

laboratory to see if the technician can tell you more than is in the report. The technician pulls you to the microscope to show you comma-shaped, gram-negative rods that he thinks look a lot like *Campylobacter* species (Figure 2).

You look up *Campylobacter* in the American Academy of Pediatrics *Red Book*® and learn that unpasteurized milk can harbor these bacteria. You also learn that *Campylobacter* species infections can mimic an acute abdomen.

Campylobacter infections usually cause diarrhea, abdominal pain, malaise, and fever. Stools may contain visible or occult blood. *Campylobacter* infections also cause mesenteric adenitis and pain. Patients with mesenteric adenitis may not have diarrhea, which makes it difficult to distinguish the condition from appendicitis. Mild infections last only 1 to 2 days and most patients recover in a week or sooner without treatment. About 20% of people with *Campylobacter* gastroenteritis relapse or have a prolonged or severe illness that can mimic acute IBD. Bacteremia, as occurred in this patient, is very uncommon.

Pseudoappendicitis sometimes is associated with *Yersinia enterocolitica* infections, which also can be acquired from contaminated milk.

Treatment

By the time *Campylobacter* gastroenteritis is diagnosed, most patients are recovering and do not benefit from antibacterial therapy. If given during the first 3 to 4 days of illness, erythromycin or azithromycin shorten the duration of symptoms. For bacteremia, treatment should be based on susceptibility tests of the isolate. *Campylobacter* species are usually susceptible to aminoglycosides, imipenem, and meropenem.

Keep in Mind

Campylobacter infections can be followed by immune-mediated complications including Guillain-Barré syndrome, Miller Fisher syndrome, Reiter syndrome, and erythema nodosum.

Chapter 48

Black, Crusty Ulcer

Presentation

One of your teenaged patients spent the summer with his grandparents in Zimbabwe, where he had the opportunity to learn about traditional cattle herding. As he was getting ready to return to the United States he noticed a pruritic papule on his arm that he thought was an insect bite. During his 2-day trip home, the papule enlarged and developed into an ulcer surrounded by vesicles (Figure 1). By the time he arrived at your office, the center of the lesion had developed a firm, black crust with a red, indurated margin (Figure 2). The lesion was not painful, but continued to itch. You find a couple of enlarged axillary lymph nodes that are tender to palpation. There are no other similar lesions, no evidence of vascular compromise, and no signs of systemic disease. This teen has had no minor skin trauma or major illnesses and the findings from a review of systems are negative.

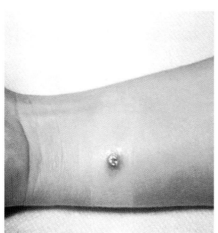

Figure 1

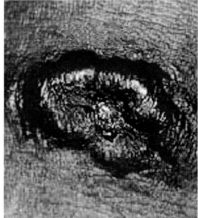

Figure 2

The description of vesicles and an ulcer lead you to ask if the insect that bit him could have been a spider. He is not even sure that he was bitten; he just assumed that the initial red bump was a bite. The black, crusted lesion with a red margin (eschar) makes you think about ecthyma gangrenosum (usually seen with *Pseudomonas aeruginosa* sepsis), but this is very unlikely in a normal host. Other organisms that can cause chancriform lesions that might look like the lesion in Figure 2 include *Treponema pallidum, Haemophilus ducreyi, Sporothrix schenckii, Bacillus anthracis, Francisella tularensis, Mycobacterium ulcerans, Mycobacterium marinum,* and *Vibrio vulnificus.* The patient denies being sexually active and the location of the lesions is not what you would expect for syphilis or chancroid. He has not been swimming at all, so *M marinum* and *V vulnificus* are unlikely. Sporotrichosis is usually associated with minor trauma to the skin and contamination with soil or plants. *M ulcerans* is endemic in areas of Australia and other tropical locations. In Australia, this infection can begin as an itchy nodule and progress to a chronic ulcer known as a Buruli ulcer. Anthrax is a zoonotic disease that is still seen in rural areas around the world. Cutaneous anthrax begins as a pruritic papule and goes on to ulcerate and form a black eschar. You suspect that this may be a spider bite and question the patient closely. Because the patient is not systemically ill and the lesion seems to be healing, you elect to observe him without treatment.

You instruct the family to return if the lesion does not continue to heal. Two days later the patient is back in your office with marked edema surrounding the eschar, increased ipsilateral axillary adenopathy, fever, malaise, and headache. Now you are concerned.

- **What does he have?**
- **How would you treat this patient?**
- **What other scenarios should you consider?**

Discussion

Diagnosis

Contact with animals or animal products infected with *Bacillus anthracis* can result in cutaneous inoculation, leading to a lesion that begins as a papule or vesicle and gets larger and ulcerates over 1 to 2 days. A black eschar forms in the center of the ulcer. The lesion may be pruritic, but is usually painless. There is usually swelling and redness around the lesion and local lymph nodes become large and painful. As long as the infection remains localized, systemic symptoms are minimal. As the infection progresses, fever, malaise, and headache become more prominent.

A Gram stain and culture should be performed on material discharged from the lesion or on a biopsy specimen if there is no discharge. If you suspect anthrax, it is best to begin antibacterial therapy before biopsy to prevent dissemination of the infection. Be sure to inform the laboratory of your clinical diagnosis to protect laboratory workers and notify local public health officials. The Centers for Disease Control and Prevention can perform additional tests and can be accessed through your local health department.

Zimbabwe is the country with the highest number of reported cases of anthrax most years and the disease occurs principally in cattle herders. There have been very few cases of naturally occurring anthrax in the United States in recent years and almost all of the cases occurred in animal handlers or mill workers. History taking for possible anthrax exposure should include asking about imported hides, hair, or wool. In today's environment of global terrorism, we also should be aware of the clinical manifestations of infections caused by agents such as anthrax that could be used as biologic weapons. In the Unites States in 2001, 22 people, including 1 infant, contracted anthrax. Most acquired the disease through contact with mail that was intentionally contaminated.

Aerosol spread seems to be the likely method that terrorists would use to infect a target population. Inhalational anthrax begins as a flu-like illness with fever, chills, cough, chest pain, muscle aches, and malaise. Within 2 to 5 days the patient develops hemorrhagic mediastinal lymphadenopathy and hemorrhagic pleural effusion; chest x-ray film may show characteristic mediastinal widening (Figure 3). By this time patients are bacteremic and toxemic with associated dyspnea, hypoxia, and shock. The nonspecific symptoms at onset, compounded by hemorrhage, edema, and necrosis caused by the 2 exotoxins produced by *B anthracis,* result in a mortality rate of about 50%.

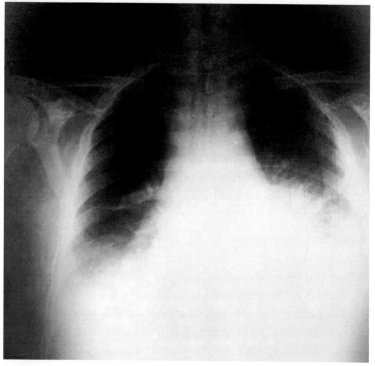

Figure 3

Anthrax can also be transmitted by the ingestion of undercooked meat. The infection can target the oropharynx, resulting in neck swelling, regional adenopathy, and sepsis, or the intestines, with severe gastroenteritis that progresses to severe abdominal pain, ascites, hematemesis, and bloody diarrhea. Like inhalation anthrax, more than half of patients die because of the rapid progression of systemic disease.

Treatment

There are no controlled studies on the treatment of anthrax and it is unlikely that there will be. Recommendations for treatment of cutaneous anthrax is ciprofloxacin for 7 to 10 days. Inhalation or ingestion anthrax should be treated with intravenous ciprofloxacin or doxycycline plus another agent with in vitro activity for at least 60 days.

Patients with disseminated cutaneous, inhalational, or gastrointestinal anthrax should be admitted to a pediatric critical care unit and managed expectantly.

Keep in Mind

B anthracis forms spores that are very stable and can travel around the world in or on animal products.

Chapter 49

Fever, Rash, Conjunctivitis, and Dizziness

Presentation

A 16-year-old young woman arrives in your office because of an abrupt onset of fever, rash, conjunctivitis, and dizziness (figures 1 and 2). Her physical examination reveals a pulse of 102 beats per minute, temperature of 38.9°C (102°F), and blood pressure of 86/50 mm Hg.

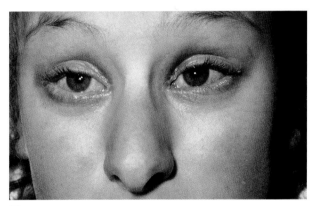

Figure 1

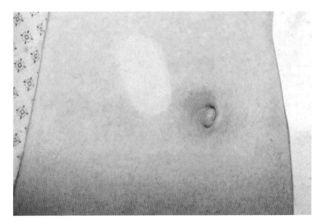

Figure 2

■ **How will you manage the care of this young woman's condition?**

■ **What is your differential diagnosis?**

■ **What information do you want?**

Discussion

Diagnosis

Without further assessment, you call emergency medical services (EMS). When the paramedics arrive, they place an intravenous line and begin fluid resuscitation. You are worried about sepsis, but do not have appropriate parenteral antibacterial agents in your office. You call the emergency department (ED) and tell them a patient is arriving by EMS and will need a bed in the pediatric intensive care unit. You tell the ED physician that you are worried about sepsis and want the patient to receive treatment for *Staphylococcus aureus, Streptococcus pyogenes* (group A β-hemolytic streptococci), *Neisseria meningitis,* and gram-negative enteric organisms.

You are also considering Kawasaki disease. She has fever, conjunctivitis, a polymorphous rash, and red hands and feet (figures 3 and 4), but the

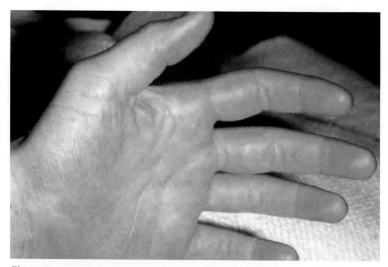

Figure 3

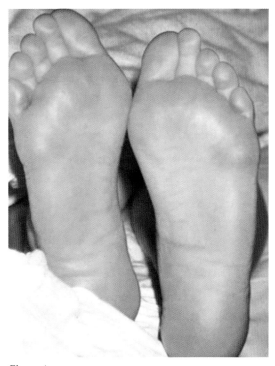

Figure 4

abrupt onset and her age make this diagnosis unlikely. You also consider whether her symptoms may be an acute presentation of systemic lupus erythematosus. Her history is negative for ill contacts, animal exposure, and travel and she is not taking any medications. Rocky Mountain spotted fever, leptospirosis, brucellosis, tularemia, and erythema multiforme drop to the bottom of your differential diagnosis.

At the hospital, the pediatric intensivist performs a comprehensive physical examination and is still unable to find anything that appears to be a primary source of infection. The intensivist notes that she has a tampon in place; the patient relates that this is the third day of her period and she has been using a superabsorbent tampon because her flow has been heavy. She uses a tampon at night.

The working diagnosis is staphylococcal toxic shock syndrome related to tampon use. The antibacterial agents that were started in the ED were nafcillin and clindamycin to treat streptococcus and staphylococcus and gentamicin to treat gram-negative enterics. The intensivist opts to continue with these agents until blood culture results are available.

The intensivist obtains appropriate laboratory tests to evaluate renal and hepatic function, a CBC and differential count (paying particular attention to the platelet count), and a creatinine phosphokinase concentration and checks for disseminated intravascular coagulation.

The laboratory tests demonstrate renal and hepatic dysfunction. You look up the case definition of staphylococcal toxic shock syndrome.

- Fever (temperature ≥38.9°C [102°F])
- Diffuse macular erythroderma
- Desquamation (1 to 2 weeks after onset, particularly palms, soles, fingers, and toes)
- Hypotension
- Involvement of 3 or more organ systems (gastrointestinal, muscular, mucous membrane, renal, hepatic, hematologic, or central nervous system)

Your patient meets the case definition for staphylococcal toxic shock syndrome.

Results from blood cultures remain negative.

Treatment
The pediatric intensivist is crucial in this situation. To prevent organ damage, the patient requires fluids to maintain adequate venous return and cardiac fill pressures. The intensivist needs to be ready to manage multisystem organ failure. Antibacterial therapy should be targeted to kill the staphylococci with a cell-wall inhibitor (nafcillin), and a second drug such as clindamycin should be administered to stop toxin production by inhibiting protein synthesis. Currently, fewer than 1% of the strains of *S aureus* associated with toxic shock syndrome are methicillin resistant. It will be important to see if this changes as community-associated methicillin-resistant *S aureus* become more prevalent. Any foreign body such as a tampon should be removed and if there is a nidus of infection, it should be drained. If the patient does not respond to several hours of aggressive antibacterial therapy, consider administering IVIG.

This patient stabilized quickly after bolus fluid and antibacterial therapy and the results of her laboratory tests returned to normal over the next few days. She was advised of the relationship between tampon use and her illness and was told that this syndrome can recur.

Keep in Mind
Be sure to measure the blood pressure of all ill patients who have diffuse erythema with or without conjunctivitis.

Desquamation usually occurs after the patient leaves the hospital; you should warn the patient that she is likely to have peeling skin on her hands, feet, fingers, or toes (figures 5 and 6).

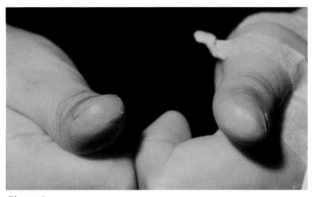

Figure 5

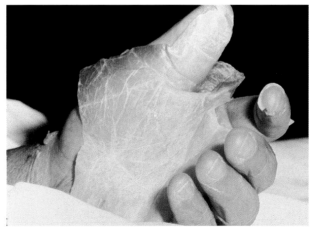

Figure 6. This is another patient with even more impressive desquamation.

Chapter 50

Sore Throat and Headache

Presentation

This teenager arrives in your office because of a headache and sore throat. Her throat is so sore she doesn't want to swallow her saliva (Figure 1). Her temperature is 38.9°C (102°F) and she has anterior cervical lymph node enlargement. You cannot palpate her spleen. The remainder of her physical examination is unremarkable.

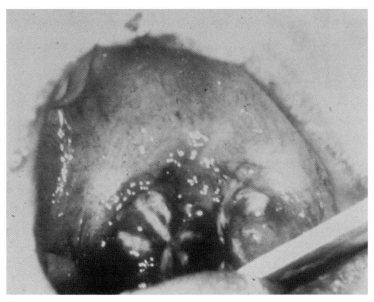

Figure 1

You suspect this teenager has group A β-hemolytic streptococcal (GABS) infection of the throat and request a rapid strep test. The negative result may be a false negative, so you send a throat swab for culture. You also decide to perform a monospot test, which also is negative. Still thinking this is GABS and wanting to speed the girl's recovery, you prescribe amoxicillin and tell the family you will let them know the culture results tomorrow.

The next day the patient returns to the office before you have a chance to call and say that the throat culture finding is negative. She does not feel any better and now has a rash (Figure 2).

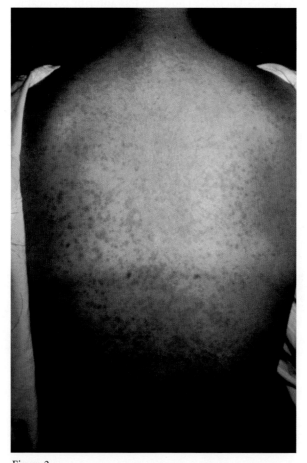

Figure 2

- ■ **What is your diagnosis?**

- ■ **Do you order any tests?**

- ■ **Do you treat this patient's condition?**

Discussion

Diagnosis

If only all of the tests we order were 100% sensitive and specific. It also would be gratifying if our clinical diagnoses were always correct. Treating with amoxicillin when you are not certain whether your patient has mononucleosis or GABS pharyngitis may cause a florid, erythematous macular rash to develop—not an acceptable method to diagnose mononucleosis.

This patient has Epstein-Barr virus (EBV) mononucleosis. Specific EBV serology done on the day she came in with the rash was positive (viral capsid antigen positive, EBV nuclear antigen negative). Heterophile antibody test (eg, monospot test) results to detect EBV mononucleosis are frequently negative in children younger than 4 years and positive in about 80% to 90% of older children and teens. Heterophile antibody test results become positive in the first 2 weeks of infection and negative over the next 6 months. In a patient with an acute onset of symptoms, the monospot test result may be negative for the first few days of infection, but often is positive after symptoms have been present for a week. The presence of atypical lymphocytosis may help establish the diagnosis of mononucleosis before the monospot test result becomes positive.

The typical manifestations of infectious mononucleosis are fever, exudative pharyngitis, cervical lymphadenopathy, malaise, and hepatosplenomegaly. Some children will have a rash with mononucleosis, but a rash is more likely and more impressive if you mistakenly give amoxicillin or other penicillins. The rash is not an allergic rash, and the pathogenesis is not known.

Treatment

Make sure you tell the patient to stop taking the amoxicillin. Infectious mononucleosis is a self-limited disease and generally is not treated. Splenomegaly occurs in nearly 80% of patients younger than 4 years and in about half of patients 4 years and older. Patients with splenomegaly should not participate in contact sports until their spleen is no longer palpable. For patients with 4+ enlarged tonsils who are having trouble swallowing or breathing, administering oral corticosteroids results in dramatic improvement, usually within 48 hours.

Corticosteroid therapy also should be considered in patients with massive splenomegaly, myocarditis, thrombocytopenia, or the hemophagocytic syndrome.

Keep in Mind

Do not treat for GABS pharyngitis unless a rapid test or throat culture result is positive. Epstein-Barr virus infection is associated with central nervous system diseases such as aseptic meningitis, encephalitis, and Guillain-Barré syndrome. Other complications of EBV infections include splenic rupture, thrombocytopenia, agranulocytosis, hemolytic anemia, hemophagocytic syndrome, orchitis, and myocarditis.

Index

Italicized page numbers denote figures.